The Newly Qualified Nurse's Survival Guide

The Newly Qualified Nurse's Survival Guide

Jackie Hole RGN, BSc (Hons)
Clinical Placement Facilitator – Clinical Placements
St Richard's Hospital, Chichester
Royal West Sussex NHS Trust

Foreword by
Sue Hopkins
Chair
RCN Practice Education Forum

Radcliffe Publishing
Oxford • Seattle

Radcliffe Publishing Ltd
18 Marcham Road
Abingdon
Oxon OX14 1AA
United Kingdom

www.radcliffe-oxford.com
Electronic catalogue and worldwide online ordering facility.

British Library Cataloguing in Publication Data

A catalogue record for this book is available from the British Library.

ISBN 1 85775 876 5

Typeset by Action Publishing Technology Ltd, Gloucester
Printed and bound by TJ International Ltd, Padstow, Cornwall

Contents

Foreword

This is truly a comprehensive, user-friendly survival guide for the newly qualified staff nurse, equating to a 'being a registered nurse for the terrified' handbook. This feels like someone is holding your hand throughout those first days of the responsibility of being a Registered Nurse at last.

Your role and responsibilities are made clear, and there is excellent guidance to help you to find out where you fit within your organisation, giving you a wider view of the targets underpinning healthcare.

In addition, there are management aspects, including delegation, objective setting, budgeting, and the book also addresses those difficult concepts like prioritisation of care and time management. There is much sensible advice about looking after yourself, making sure that you are fed and watered as well as everyone else.

The book sets you off on your journey from getting the most out of your final placement, preparing the application for a post, easing you into dealing with common clinical problems, using experts to help you, then towards becoming a mentor and gate-keeping the profession.

It is also highly recommended for more experienced nurses as a refresher to their knowledge, as it contains a wealth of fundamental practical advice about good nursing care, all in one book. One vital phrase that jumped out at me was to 'look at your patient', one of many truly practical yet essential pointers towards becoming an effective and caring professional nurse.

The examples given bring the advice to life, and the wise words are completed by a checklist so that you can see your achievements.

Good luck to you as you embark upon your career in nursing, and I hope that this becomes a well-worn text used for reference and advice for at least the first year!

Sue Hopkins
Chair
RCN Practice Education Forum
October 2004

Preface

I have been qualified as a staff nurse for 11 years. During those years I have had many experiences of good and bad nursing. It is my belief that good nursing comes from within and is not an attitude that can be learned. I feel that if you start off well in your career and learn how to nurse in a thinking and empathetic way, your patients will rcap the rewards and you will never lose those qualities. Throughout your nursing course you will have had structure and processes to follow (sometimes too much!) which have guided you to learn the appropriate skills and gain the knowledge required to become a staff nurse. However, once qualified this structure all but disappears and you can feel 'abandoned'.

My background is mainly within medical nursing, where I managed to reach the dizzy heights of ward manager. Following this and having always wanted to be involved in clinical education, I obtained the post of clinical placement facilitator. My remit was to ensure an excellent learning environment within my NHS Trust – the Royal West Sussex NHS Trust in Chichester. This role meant that I was often in close contact with newly qualified nurses. I felt that they lacked direction and needed to know that they were not alone. It was for these reasons I decided to write this book. I hope that you find it useful and enjoy reading it.

Jackie Hole
October 2004

About the author

When do you know that you want to be a nurse?

For me, it was when I was still at school. I can't actually remember thinking, yes, I want to go into nursing, but I knew I wanted to look after people. Originally I thought I wanted to be a children's Nanny. I went to College to train, but soon realised that I wanted more than that. The course that I did enabled me to experience all sorts of caring skills and I was then able to identify that nursing was what suited me best.

I worked in a Nursing Home at weekends and learnt how to give good fundamental care. I applied to do a Pre-Registration Nursing course at three schools of nursing.

My first interview was unsuccessful and I thought it was the end of the world – it was all I wanted to do. I knew that I couldn't give up and that I would make a good nurse. I went to my second interview and was offered a place in Chichester. I am now glad – it was fate – I made some lifelong friends and was fortunate to train in an excellent Trust, and I still work there to this day.

Once qualified, I realised that Medicine was where I wanted to make my career. I progressed and soon reached the position of Senior Staff Nurse. I also realised that I wanted to teach, and decided to undertake a BSc (Hons) in Health Studies. Following this I obtained a Ward Manager's post on an Acute Admissions ward.

My present position was then advertised and I was offered the post, following a successful interview. (During this time I also got married and had two wonderful children!) This post has enabled me to facilitate and develop the learning environment within the Trust and has allowed me to enjoy both clinical and managerial aspects of nursing. I am currently undertaking an MA in Higher Education to allow me to become a Practice Educator within the clinical environment.

My philosophy?

This is what I believe, and I try to apply these principles every day.

- Nursing comes from within. In order to be a good nurse you must give something of yourself every day.
- Every patient deserves your best care, no matter how you are feeling or what is happening in your life.
- Always care for patients and their families as you would wish to be cared for. Put yourself in their place.
- Pay attention to the details. These are the things that matter most to patients.
- Always ask questions and remember that you can learn something from every situation.
- Think positive and keep your sense of humour.

Introduction

After three years of training, I thought I was ready to become a staff nurse, but now I feel scared that I don't know enough.

Almost all of the newly qualified nurses with whom I have come into contact feel this way to varying degrees.

Having once been newly qualified myself, and now supporting those who are in the clinical environment, I feel that these nurses need something to guide them through this difficult but exciting time. This book aims to provide a realistic, helpful and sometimes comic look at post-student life. It will also help to soften the 'reality shock', as described by Patricia Benner (1984), that newly qualified nurses can feel. They have a sometimes unrealistic or 'fairytale' image of what being a qualified nurse is all about, and while they are students they are often protected by their mentor from the stresses and problems that can arise.

The first chapter looks at how it feels to be finishing three years of intensive training, and guides you through what you should be doing in order to prepare yourself for being newly qualified. The following chapters and the objectives contained within them will help to give some structure to your first year as a staff nurse.

I hope that you enjoy the book and find it helpful and supportive. The comical anecdotes along the way will help you to realise that everyone has felt the same and experienced similar situations. Above all, enjoy it!

1

Pre-qualification

Use the time during your management/supervised practice placement to really look at the areas in which you are lacking practical knowledge. For some, it may be as simple as not having inserted very many catheters. For others, it may be the whole management experience that is daunting. Try to work with the person in charge of the ward as much as possible to gain experience in how others manage a group or a ward of patients. Request that you actually take charge under their guidance, so that you experience what it is like to really manage the ward. It is a good idea to work with more than one person in order to see different leadership styles in action. You can then pick out the approaches that suit you.

This may be the point at which you decide which speciality you want to start work in, or you may still have no idea about this. If that is the case, perhaps a rotational contract would be best for you so that you can find out where your area of interest lies. You will find that most NHS Trusts offer rotational posts for newly qualified nurses. They will run over varying lengths of time, but two years is an ideal period. This will give you the chance to experience medicine, surgery and high dependency care. Each Trust will manage this differently – the placements may be set from the beginning or flexible to allow the programme to fit individual needs. This is a really good way of finding out what suits you and what you enjoy the most, and it will also provide excellent experience. Many nurses find that they are ready for a more senior position following the completion of a rotation programme.

Use the following to guide you through your last placement to ensure that you get the maximum benefit from the experience.

Management/supervised practice placement objectives

The following are designed to enhance the objectives set for you by your university. They include both the theoretical and practical aspects of the last placement.

This is one of the most important placements of your training. It is during this placement that you will have the opportunity to consolidate the skills and knowledge you have acquired during your training. Make the most of the opportunity and remember that this is your last chance to 'practise' your skills before you become a staff nurse. If you feel that there are still certain skills or gaps in your knowledge that you have missed out on throughout your training, now is the time to make sure you address those issues. As well as ensuring that you have accrued all of the necessary skills, the following will help to guide you through the management process.

These are the skills that you will be using once you are qualified, so use this time to practise them as much as possible. This will make the transition from student to staff nurse much easier.

Allocation and delegating skills

Practise allocating staff to patients. This will be much less difficult while you are a student. Once you are qualified you will be expected to do this, and it is important to practise how to get it right. For example, you will need to find out who has been on duty the shift before, as you will want to provide continuity for your patients. You may need to find out which staff are in which team, if that is the way the ward is organised. You may also need to enquire as to how long the staff are on duty. Whether they are on a long or short shift may influence where you allocate them. If you need to allocate a registered nurse and an unqualified nurse to each group of patients, you will want to ensure that one of them at least is working a long shift so that someone knows about those patients throughout the day. This will ensure that even fairly simple matters, such as what a particular patient has eaten that day, are not neglected.

It is also important to remember that, when allocating staff, you may encounter negative comments such as 'Oh no! Not that patient again today!' These kind of comments are difficult to deal with, so the more practice you have in doing so the better. It is essential that this type of judgemental attitude *is* challenged and not allowed to continue unchecked. This type of communication is very damaging, as is well documented by Stockwell (1972), and it can cause negative feelings towards the patient before the nurse has even met them. Ways of challenging this behaviour include pointing out what you like about the patient or pointing out why you think they may behave in a certain way. Otherwise, the more this negative type of attitude is allowed to continue unchallenged, the more negative the team becomes.

'It's not what you say, it's the way that you say it'

Delegation is another area where newly qualified staff experience huge difficulties. Often they do not feel confident enough to ask someone else to do something for them. Consequently, they try to do all of the work themselves and end up leaving late or providing less than adequate standards of care. Other members of staff will not mind if you delegate tasks to them, so long as you apply these basic rules:

* Is it something they are competent to do? When delegating, you remain responsible for that care if you do not delegate appropriately as stated in the Code of Professional Conduct (Nursing and Midwifery Council 2002).
* Have you explained clearly what it is you want them to do and why?
* Are you genuinely busy yourself, or is it just something that you do not want to do?

As long as you ask the other member of staff in a courteous manner and stick to these rules, there will be few problems. That said, there may always be someone who has the potential to react in a negative way to your request. These people are often known for this type of behaviour and it should be dealt with swiftly by their manager. If you experience this type of reaction, try discussing the matter with the member of staff, or if you do not feel confident enough to do this, talk to your manager.

Management of a group of patients

This is something that can be practised well during your supervised practice placement. It is important to know about each of your patients, including their care needs, social situation, relatives and medical plan. You must find out this information quickly once you are on duty. Some of it may become apparent during the handover, but the rest can be found out by reading the nursing and medical notes and talking to your patients. Start the shift by making a list of things that need to be done. This list may well start during handover. This way you will ensure that you do not forget to do something important, and it also is very satisfying to be able to cross the items off your list as you go along. If you do have unfinished tasks on your list at the end of your shift, you can then hand them over to the next shift of nurses. Remember that nursing is a 24-hour profession – you don't need to get everything completed during your shift. However, you do need to ensure that you have prioritised your list and that the essential jobs have been completed.

If you are responsible for a side room as well as a bay of patients, try to go and say hello to them first. It is important that you greet your patients and introduce yourself to them before you do anything else. If you get stuck on the drug round or with doctors, you may not see the patients in side rooms until well into the shift. Patients, especially those in side rooms, may feel neglected or uncertain who is looking after them that day if they have not seen you.

You must ensure that you work as part of a team. You will need to know about the care needs of all of your patients so that you can discuss with the nurse you are working with which of you will do what. You cannot expect the unqualified nurse to perform all of the essential care for your patients. Not only is this unfair, but it also means that you will not be seeing pressure areas, communicating with your patients, assessing their nutritional needs or teaching and being a role model for the untrained staff. It is all too easy to get caught up in paperwork, telephone conversations and referrals. Do they all need to be done as a priority, or can some of these things wait until the patient care has been done?

It is important to realise what is going on in the rest of the ward. It is very easy to become isolated in your bay. Make sure that you are aware of potential problems in other bays, and don't forget to offer help if it is required. You would not be expected to know everything about all of the patients on the ward, but you need to know about acutely ill patients, violent patients, etc., in case your assistance is required. If a colleague is caring for such a patient, remember to make sure that they are coping with the situation, and offer your help. They may well have more experience and knowledge than you with regard to this type of situation, but your support will be much appreciated. Think how you would feel in the same situation. You may also learn the best way to deal with these issues.

Doctors' rounds and case conferences

Doctors' rounds, especially when the consultant is present, can be very daunting when you are newly qualified. While you are on your final placement attend as many of these rounds as you can. Watch what your mentor does – how he/she interacts with the doctors, the sort of questions that are asked and how he/she fields questions that he/she does not know the answer to. Once you feel confident enough, you may be able to attend these rounds without your mentor. As long as you know what has happened to that patient over the past 24–48 hours, what their social situation is like and what nursing care they are currently requiring, you should be able to answer most of their questions. It is very important that a nurse is present on these rounds. The reason for this is not to fuel the doctors' egos or just because they want a nurse there. It is because you can provide valuable information about your patients. You are the one who knows them best. The doctors will only see their patients for a few minutes each day. You are there as their advocate and as someone who knows exactly how they will be able to manage at home. You will also know if there are problems with relatives or accommodation. The patient will feel more comfortable with you there, and may well feel more confident and able to communicate. Most patients consider doctors to be quite formidable and that 'doctor knows best', so they may not question plans that are made at the end of their bed. You will be able to make sure that the patient understands what is being said and is in agreement with it.

You will be able to provide the same valuable role during a case conference. As the person who has probably had the most contact with the relatives, you will be able to pass on information about the home situation and family dynamics. This will help to ensure a more effective discharge.

Drug rounds

Try to gain as much experience of these as you can during this placement. Once you are qualified, many Trusts will require you to undertake a drug assessment before you are deemed competent to perform drug rounds independently. Some universities have also written this into their curriculum so that a student must pass a drug assessment before they can qualify. This helps to ensure that both you and your manager are confident that you are competent. The more practice you have as a student, the more confident you will feel. Try to perform at least one drug round per shift. It is important that you actually dispense and administer the drugs under supervision. You will not learn if you are only observing. You may feel guilty about taking up too much of your mentor's time, as you are bound to be much slower than they are. However, they understand that in order for you to be confident, you must practise, so don't be afraid to negotiate this with them. The more you do, the more efficient you will become. This is also an excellent way of learning about the more common drugs, their usage and side-effects.

Find out the answers to the following questions.

- What should I do if I disagree with a prescription?
- What should I do if the prescription is illegible?
- What should I do if I make a mistake? What is the Trust policy?
- How do I order drugs out of pharmacy hours?
- What should I do if I can't give a drug for some reason?
- What drugs am I not allowed to give?

Off-duty planning and staffing issues

Although it is unlikely that you will be required to actually write the off duty, it is important that you understand the intricacies of staff planning. Ask the ward manager to explain to you how they go about deciding what shifts everyone will be working. They may feel that it is appropriate for you to try writing it yourself. This is an excellent way to learn how difficult this task is! It will also help you to appreciate that you can never please everyone! You will gain an insight into what staffing levels should be in order for the ward to be considered a safe environment and what can be done if it isn't. Skill mix is another consideration when planning the off duty. You must ensure that there is someone competent to take charge of the ward and that there are enough qualified staff to undertake the care of the patients. There must also be enough unqualified staff to assist with the essential care of the patients. Sometimes it is necessary to review the skill mix or staffing levels. For example, a patient may be very acutely unwell and require one-to-one nursing. In this case extra help must be found. Find out what the options are in this situation.

Find out what happens if a member of staff is not performing as they should or is giving cause for concern. What is the Trust policy? Talk to the ward manager about what they expect of a newly qualified nurse. This may differ depending on the area in which the manager works. Generally the issues will be based on the following common principles:

- working in accordance with the Nursing and Midwifery Council (NMC) Code of Conduct
- respect for other members of staff. This means valuing all members of the team and their contribution to patient care. Their opinions and beliefs may not be the same as yours, but this adds to the richness of the experience and the complexity of the team

- someone who is aware of their own limitations and can identify areas that require development
- a member of staff who is empathetic and caring towards their patients and their families
- an expectation that the nurse will work to the best of their abilities and be committed to high standards of care.

Ordering of supplies

Find out where supplies come from. For example, drug supplies come from a different department to catheters. Ensure that you know how to order more supplies if stocks are low or if you should suddenly run out of something. Do you know who to contact and where? How do they arrive on the ward? Who is responsible for unpacking and ensuring that they are safely stored?

Use of the computer

The computer is being used more and more within clinical areas. Some Trusts have all of their nursing documentation available on computer, and some use electronic prescribing. All Trusts encourage evidence-based practice, so use of the Internet and libraries is actively encouraged. Some wards will have access to the Internet on the ward computer, while in others you may need to use the Trust library facilities.

You will need to know how to input patient data, and you will need to access a Trust training course. It is very important that patient details are recorded accurately to ensure that the most up-to-date information is known about the patient, and for reasons such as auditing, costing and statistics.

Sister's meetings

If these are held, try to go along with the Sister of your ward. These are formal, informative gatherings of the sisters within a certain directorate (e.g. medicine). At these meetings, information and good practice are shared and managers have the opportunity to share information with each other and then disseminate this to their ward staff. These meetings also provide an opportunity for managers to support each other and provide a network to work within. You will get the chance to observe the dynamics within the group and to see how problems are shared and acted upon. This is a very powerful group of people who can identify risk issues and change practice.

Knowledge of policies and procedures

Find out where to gain information about nursing, health and safety and human resources policies. Ward areas should have copies of these for you to see. You would not be expected to know every policy inside out, but you would be expected to have read them and know where to locate them. You need to know which are the most important ones – ask your mentor.

Important points to remember when looking for a job

There are a number of things to look out for when considering a post as a newly qualified staff nurse.

- Think about the travelling time to and from work. You may be working long shifts, so you probably don't want to add more than half an hour's travel on to this. Especially at the beginning, you will find that you will become extremely tired due to the high amounts of physical and mental energy you will be using.

- Take notice of a Trust's reputation. If it is well known for looking after its staff, this is the kind of place in which you want to start your career. This will mean that you will be well supported. Ask for an informal visit before your interview. A good Trust will invest the time to arrange this for you. When you go for your visit, look at how staff communicate with each other. Do they say hello when they pass each other in the corridors? Do people look happy? Does the hospital look clean and well cared for? What sort of reception do you get when you are introduced to staff? Are they welcoming and friendly? Do the wards seem calm and well organised? All of these will give you a clue to what it would be like to work there. Also ask about support for newly qualified nurses.
  - Do they provide a supernumerary period?
  - Is there a pre-set programme for you to follow?
  - What post-registration training is available?
  - Do they provide a rotational programme?
  - Is there someone within the Trust who supports newly qualified nurses?
- Ask for an informal visit with the ward manager whose ward you are applying for before the interview. This will be an advantage for two reasons. First, you will see the ward where you could be working and you may meet some of your potential colleagues. You will have the chance to ask questions about the type of patients who are cared for. Secondly, the ward manager will get to meet you before the interview, when you will be less nervous. This will give a good first impression, so try to be keen and enthusiastic.
- Visit the Trust website. This will give you an impression of what the Trust values as important. Remember that some

websites may not be up to date, so the vacancies page may not be a true reflection of the availability of jobs. You should be able to view recent Healthcare Commission visit reports and other information that will tell you more about the Trust.

Interview skills

You should take along to the interview:

- your portfolio
- your CV.

What will happen at the interview?

When you arrive, the interviewers will introduce themselves. There will probably be just two people on the panel for most junior staff nurse posts. The panel members are most likely to be the ward manager of the ward on which you have applied for a job and their senior staff nurse, another ward manager or someone from the human resources department. They may tell you what the interview will involve. Each panel member will then ask you their set of questions. At the end, they may ask to see your portfolio or CV. They may well look at it there and then, or they may ask if they can look at it and return it to you at a later date. They may ask you where you will be later in the day so that they can inform you of the outcome of the interview. Sometimes they cannot do this, and they may then say that they will let you know the next day or in writing. The way they let you know does not mean anything in terms of whether you have got the job or not. It may just mean that they are waiting for references or are interviewing again the next day. You will be asked whether you have any questions for them. Try to have a few questions prepared to ask, as this shows that you are interested and brings the interview to a natural close. The interview will probably take about half an hour.

Handy hints

- Remember to keep smiling.
- If you don't understand a question, ask the interviewer to repeat it or rephrase it – don't try to bluff your way through it!
- Try to speak at a normal rate, and try not to rush your answers.
- Take a silent deep breath before answering a question, and think about your answer.
- Look at the person who is directing the question to you. Maintain eye contact.
- Try to look smart and professional.
- Wear something you feel comfortable in.
- Sell yourself!
- Practise beforehand with a friend. The more you say the answers out loud, the better it will sound in the interview.
- Read around subjects that the interviewers are likely to ask you about – for example *The Essence of Care* (Department of Health 2001). It will come across in the interview if you have done some pre-interview reading and preparation.
- Shake hands when you enter the room, even if you know the interviewers. Practise your handshake! This may not be something that you have done much in the past, and it makes an impression on the interviewer. A firm handshake suggests confidence, whereas a 'limp' handshake seems to suggest submissiveness or low self-esteem.
- Make sure that you eat something beforehand, even if you don't feel like it. It will give your brain some energy and stop your stomach rumbling!

What will they ask?

The following questions are for guidance only and may or may not be asked. Be prepared for other questions to come up as well.

- Tell me why you want to be a nurse.
- What did you enjoy most about your training?
- In which area of nursing do you feel most confident?
- What are your strengths?
- What are your weaknesses?
- What do you think you will be doing in five years' time?
- What do you know about recent Government/Department of Health reports?
- Tell me about the NHS Plan.
- What would you do if someone asked you to do something you were not sure about?
- What would you do if a consultant questioned your practice?
- Tell me about yourself.
- How do you feel that your role will change when you become a staff nurse?
- Is there anything that worries you about becoming a staff nurse?
- How do you feel about delegating tasks to healthcare assistants (HCAs) or students?

What shouldn't I do?

- Don't lie! It is obvious if you try to bluff your way out of a question. If you don't know the answer, say so. Ask the interviewer to tell you more about it. Try saying 'Sorry, I don't know much about that – could you tell me more about it?' This sounds much better than 'I don't know'.

- Don't look at the same person all the time. It is very off-putting if you are asked a question by one person and you then reply to someone else!
- Don't try to make a fashion statement at your interview!
- Don't look a mess!
- Don't try to outsmart your interviewer. You may come off looking worse.
- Don't keep looking out of the window.
- Don't worry! Try to enjoy it.

CV writing and application forms

When compiling your CV, remember that potential employers will probably not be interested in what you did before your training, unless this was nursing related.

It is quite acceptable to start your CV with a summary of your training. The first page should start with a brief summary of who you are. This should then be followed by your experience, starting with the most recent. When writing this part, try to highlight areas that you had responsibility for – for example, you may have acted as a link nurse. You can also list any achievements or innovations in which you were involved – for example, you may have been included in some Essence of Care work in a clinical area. All of these will make you stand apart from other newly qualified staff, whose CVs will all look very similar at this point in their career.

Your application form is very important. This is the first impression that you will be giving to a potential employer. In order to maximise your chances of being short-listed, ensure that you complete the form as fully as possible. Fill it in first in pencil, to minimise mistakes. When you come to the part where you are asked to write about yourself, practise this on a spare sheet of paper. This is where you must sell yourself and make the employer want to interview you. Remember to keep a copy of what you have written, as there may be a considerable time gap between completing the form and having your interview. The interviewers may ask you about what you have written, so read through your copy the day before.

Ensure that the people you indicate as references are relevant and recent. Most employers will expect to see cited as referees on a newly qualified nurse's application form a tutor and a ward manager or senior staff nurse from a recent placement. Ensure that you have asked their permission to include them as a referee. It is not good etiquette for the reference to be called for without the referee's prior knowledge of the possibility of a request. Some people will actually throw the request straight in the bin if this happens, so be warned!

Portfolio building

A portfolio is a record of a nurse's achievements and experience. It is a requirement of the Nursing and Midwifery Council, and from 1998 all nurses can be called upon to submit their portfolio and provide evidence of relevant study over three years (Nursing and Midwifery Council 2001). The portfolio should not be looked upon as a chore, but as something that can help you to consolidate what you have done and be beneficial to you. For example, when applying for a job it can be the difference between getting the job or not! It shows the interviewer that you have made an effort and demonstrates exactly what you can offer. It is helpful for the interview panel if you can let them have your portfolio a couple of days before the interview so that they have time to look at it properly. This also gives the impression of an organised and efficient person.

This is not a comprehensive guide to compiling a portfolio, as there are many different packages available on the market.

However, the nurse can easily compile his/her own portfolio at a fraction of the cost and can usually produce a more comprehensive file that combines the best parts from the other packages.

The following is a guide to the various parts of a portfolio.

- The curriculum vitae should include:
  - name and address
  - a short summary of yourself
  - career history – starting with the most recent history, and including a brief summary of responsibilities held
  - education history and qualifications
  - professional training and PIN number
  - short courses
  - long courses
  - personal section
  - interests.
- Your personal nursing philosophy should include:
  - the care you provide to your patients
  - your aims
  - how you achieve your aims
  - the environment that you wish to provide.
- Personal objectives should include:
  - short-term objectives
  - long-term objectives.
- Reflection on past experience should include:
  - each nursing job you have held
  - the skills you have gained from each job.
    1 What practical and clinical skills have you become competent in?
    2 How have you extended your knowledge and understanding?
    3 How have you developed with regard to moral and ethical decision making?

- Current job description.
- Professional courses should include:
  - short courses
  - long courses
  - a short description of each course and what you gained from attending it.
- Teaching experience should include:
  - teaching sessions you have held
  - a short description of the session and who it was aimed at.
- Reflective diary. This is personal and need not be submitted if your portfolio is asked for by the Nusing and Midwifery Council. It should include reflections on incidents and situations and what you have learned from them. A good model of reflective practice that can be used is that of Gibbs (1988).

2

Post-qualification: the first few weeks

So you've found your ideal job, been for the interview and got the post! Well done! But what now?

You may feel that you need a short break between completing your training and commencing your new post as a staff nurse. If you feel this way, negotiate with your ward manager, as this would not usually be a problem. Do remember, though, that they may be keeping the job open for you for a few months due to the fact that they need to wait for you to complete your training.

When you begin your job, you may be supernumerary for the first few weeks. This will enable you to ease gently into your new role under the supervision of another trained nurse. You may feel that you just want to 'get on' with being responsible for your own patients, but make the most of this time – it will never happen again and it can be very useful! Use the time to find out about the documentation used, the processes that work within the Trust and the team dynamics. Ask lots of questions and use the objectives on the following pages to guide you. Don't try to learn everything within a few weeks. This will probably be the biggest learning curve you are likely to experience in the whole of your career. And don't forget that even nurses who have been qualified for 20 years don't know everything – we all learn something new every day. That's the best part of being a nurse – every day is different!

Your first day

It's your first day as a staff nurse!

How do you feel?

- Self-conscious – you're in a staff nurse uniform, yet you feel like an impostor ('The other staff nurses deserve their uniforms'). Of course all newly qualified nurses feel like this. You can't quite believe that you are wearing that long-awaited uniform, the uniform you have seen others wearing and thought you'd never get! Reassure yourself – you do deserve it! You've spent three years getting here, you've worked incredibly hard, you may have encountered bad mentors and placements at times, you've sacrificed nights out to study (or maybe not!) and you've scrimped to buy your supper. Wear that uniform with pride – it's what you've been longing for. The first time you walk down the ward and a patient calls out to you 'staff nurse!', it's a great feeling – you have arrived!

- Nervous – everyone feels this way. 'Will I know enough?', 'What if I look stupid?' and 'What if I do something wrong?' The staff will be expecting you to be nervous and anxious. They will support you and make sure that you are looked after. You should be assigned a mentor. If this is not forthcoming, ask.

- Unconfident – you will probably feel as if you don't know enough at this point. You will not be expected to know everything. Be honest, and talk to the staff on duty – they have all been there. Once you have settled into the shift and started talking to your patients, you will begin to relax. Make sure that you understand what is expected of you, and ask for clarification if necessary. At the end of your first day you will be feeling much better and looking forward to the next shift.

- On your own – for the past three years you have been part

of a group of fellow students and have become especially good friends with a number of them. You may feel that you have reached the end of an era and that everything has changed. If there are newly qualified support groups on offer, try to go along to them. You will have the chance to meet up with your old friends and maybe make some new ones! Remember that it's the start of a *new* era, and that soon you will make friends within your ward or department and feel more at home.

During your first shift make sure that you find out about the ward environment. During a quiet moment ask a member of staff to show you around the ward and the rest of the hospital. Find out where the following departments are: salaries and wages, human resources, the nurse bank office, hospital chapel, chapel of rest, porters' base, theatres, recovery area, ITU, high-dependency unit, coronary care, medical assessment unit, Accident and Emergency, medical records, outpatients, pharmacy, X-ray, pathology and the emergency drug cupboard.

By the end of your first day on the ward, make sure that you know about the following.

Cardiac arrest procedures

- Where is the equipment kept? This would usually be in a designated place on the ward that is easily accessible. It is important that the equipment is always kept in the same place so that all staff can locate it quickly.
- What equipment would be required in an emergency situation? The Crash Trolley will include the necessary equipment for airway management, intubation, peripheral and central venous access devices, fluids, and venepuncture equipment. The emergency drugs, which will be sealed

until they are required, will include drugs such as atropine, bicarbonate and adrenaline. With regard to emergency suction, most wards will have wall suction at each bed, but if a patient requires emergency treatment in a bathroom, for example, this may be needed. The defibrillator may be a manual or advisory machine. Nurses can train to use an advisory defibrillator and must update their training annually.

- All emergency equipment should be checked by a trained nurse once a day to ensure that it is working correctly and that it is all there. Fluids and other expiry-sensitive equipment must be checked to ensure that they have not passed their expiry date.

- Find out how to summon the Crash Team. This will usually be via the switchboard, who will then bleep the team. There will also be a procedure for summoning a particular doctor in an emergency, often called 'fast bleeping'.

- What would your role be in a crash situation? As a newly qualified nurse you would not be expected to take charge of the arrest, even if the patient was one of your allocated patients. If this was the case, you would be expected to know what had happened to your patient immediately before the arrest. Your role would then be to assist the team in any way in which you felt confident. This may be assisting with the emergency drugs, passing equipment to the medics from the crash trolley, setting up the defibrillator and cardiac leads, recording an ECG, obtaining a set of vital signs, assisting the anaesthetist in maintaining the patient's airway, performing chest compressions or just observing the arrest. This is quite acceptable if you have not had much experience in emergency situations. Try to find somewhere to stand where you can see what is happening but where you are not in the way – next to the anaesthetist is usually a good place. Try not to end up with the job of the 'runner' (the person who is asked to go and find the equipment or drugs that are required which are not immediately to hand). As a newly qualified nurse you will probably not know what they are, or where to find them, which would be incredibly stressful. I can remember when I was first qualified, and during an arrest I was asked to go to ITU for a piece of equipment. By the time I arrived in ITU, I had forgotten what the doctors had asked for! I had to ring the ward and ask the person who answered the phone to go and ask the crash team what it was that they wanted! This was obviously *very* embarrassing! Needless to say, I did not volunteer to be the runner again until I was much more experienced. If it is one of your patients who has arrested, you should ring the next of kin as soon as possible. It is not a good idea to tell them over the phone that the patient has arrested, or that they have died, if that is the case, especially if the relative is elderly. The last thing you want is a collapsed relative on the end of the phone. Tell them that their relative has taken a 'turn for the worse' or has 'collapsed', and ask them to come to the ward as soon as possible. Ensure that you or someone else arranges that they are met at the entrance to the ward, as you will not want them to walk into the arrest situation.

Fire evacuation and procedures

- Look around the ward and find out where the fire extinguishers and break-glass points are.
- Find out what the procedure is if fire is suspected.
- Find out where you should evacuate the patients to if necessary. Sometimes this is outside, or it may be the next fire 'compartment' (this may be the next ward or department).
- Where are your emergency exits? Are they accessible? If

they are blocked by equipment, ensure that you talk to the nurse in charge and move it to a more appropriate place.

Over the next few weeks find out about...

Case conferences

If your ward holds regular case conferences, go along to a few with another staff nurse. You will gain an idea of what your future role will be within these meetings. Observe who usually leads the meeting and the sort of questions they may ask you. These will often be about the social situation of the patient and their progress with regard to the discharge plan.

Taking charge of your group of patients

As you are probably still supernumerary, you will be working alongside another staff nurse. Use this opportunity to take charge of your group of patients under the supervision of someone else. Negotiate with them the areas in which you are confident and those where you are less confident, and ask them to assist you with these areas. It will be comforting to know that you have someone to call upon, but that they are not looking over your shoulder all the time. Make the most of this opportunity as it will never happen again!

Fundamental nursing care

Think about the fundamental nursing care that you will need to provide for your group of patients. This is really something you know plenty about, and you should feel confident in doing it following your three years of training. Think about the care in a holistic way, and about who you want to provide that care. All too often the HCA/student is providing this care without the support and guidance of a qualified nurse. It is very important that you actively participate in this alongside them so that you can lead the care given, role model and teach. *The Essence of Care* (Department of Health 2001) provides nurses with a tool to benchmark their practice and improve that practice. It also encourages the sharing of good practice and networking across wards and Trusts. This important document reinforces and reminds us of what *patients* say is important, and of the fundamentals of our role. There are nine elements:

1 Communication – that it, thinking about how we communicate with patients, staff and relatives. Is our communication effective? Can patients and relatives understand what they are being told? How do we communicate (verbally, in writing, non-verbally, electronically)? What would your patient like to be called?

2 Personal and oral hygiene. Ask yourself whether you provide this fully. Think about when you are providing a 'bed bath'. Do you take off the patient's anti-embolism stockings and wash their legs and feet? Do you ensure the skin's integrity by applying moisturiser if required? Do you provide *regular* oral hygiene or is it just given once a day? Ensure that you provide a sputum pot for those patients who require one. Do you make sure that the patient has the opportunity to wash their hands after using the commode/toilet? When you have finished washing your patient do you tidy up the area and change the bed linen?

3 Privacy and dignity. Think about the person, not the patient. Do they like to wear make-up? Do they really need to be in nightwear, especially on a rehabilitation ward? Have you closed the curtains properly and do you keep going in and out because you've forgotten something? Do people constantly come behind the curtains to ask you

questions while the patient is undressed? How is confidentiality maintained in your area? How do staff talk about patients during handover? Do they use derogatory terms? Is this challenged?

4   Pressure areas. What pressure-relieving devices do you have available? Are they adequate and are there enough of them? How regularly do you provide pressure-area care and when is it assessed? Think about why patients develop pressure ulcers. Is there anything you can do to improve this?

5   Safety. What risk-management structure is in place? How do you assess risk? What happens when a risk is identified? Are patients easily identifiable? What policies are in place to ensure patient safety? How are confused patients cared for? Do staff know about the Mental Health Act?

6   Self-care. What do you do to encourage self-care? Why is it so important? What happens to patients if this is not encouraged?

7   Nutrition. How do you assess and monitor your patient's nutritional needs? What barriers are there to patients being fed adequately? What can be done about those barriers? How can working with the patient's family help? Do you make sure that the environment is conducive to eating and drinking? Can the patient reach the food and drink? Is there a full urinal on their table?! Do you make a conscious effort to take the patient to the bathroom at mealtimes, rather than making them use the commode by the bed? Make sure that you offer the patient the opportunity to wash their hands before meals.

8   Bowel and bladder care. What processes are in place to monitor bowel and bladder problems? Are the solutions to these problems evidence based? What facilities are available in your area? Are the patients encouraged to self-care? Is the call bell always within reach?

9   Record keeping. What documents are used and where are

they kept? Are they relevant and kept up to date? Who writes in them and are these individuals adequately trained? Do they enable good and continuous patient care? Who has access to records? What do you know about data protection and confidentiality?

When looking at the above elements, ask yourself the following questions.

1 What do we do as a team that is really good practice?
2 How can we share that good practice with other wards/departments/Trusts?
3 What do we do that could be improved?
4 What do other wards/departments/Trusts do?
5 How can we go about improving it?
6 How can we implement the change in practice and disseminate our work?

Undertaking a ward round

- This will be daunting even if you have attended many ward rounds as a student. It will become an altogether different experience now that you have your staff-nurse uniform on. Doctors will not necessarily know that you are newly qualified unless your hospital has some way of identifying this (e.g. epaulettes or a different badge). This may be more difficult if you were a mature student, as other staff may assume that you have been qualified for some time.
- You will be expected to know the answers to certain questions. If you don't know the patients very well, look at the nursing notes beforehand. It is a good idea to find out when the rounds are likely to take place so that you can be well prepared. The information that the doctors

are likely to want will concern the patient's social situation, what nursing care they currently require and how they have been in the last 24 hours. For example, if the patient has been admitted with chest pain, the doctors are going to want to know if the patient has reported any pain and, if so, what relieved it.

- Make notes as you go along, as you may forget what was said afterwards. There is no reason why you can't take the nursing notes along with you – this will help you to find the answers to questions that the doctors are likely to ask. If you don't know about the social situation, for example, say so and ask the patient if they are able to answer the question. Doctors sometimes forget that patients can answer for themselves! If the patient can't give them an answer, then say that you will talk to the relatives and let them know. You can't be expected to know everything about all of your patients, but if you are well prepared you will know most of the information about them.

- Try to attend *all* doctors' rounds if you can. This will not always be possible due to the workload that day. If you can't go, make sure that you find out what was said as soon as possible, either by asking them at the end or by looking in the medical notes. For example, they may forget to tell you that they want an infusion discontinued, and if you don't look at the notes until a few hours later, the patient may receive drugs that they did not require or that are no longer being prescribed for them. It is very important to attend if possible, so that not only can you provide essential information and act as the patient's advocate, but also you can go back and check with the patient that they have understood what has been said. Often they will not say that they don't understand when the doctors are there, so you must ensure that they are aware of what is happening and provide an explanation if necessary.

Patient admission

- If you are starting work in the hospital in which you trained, this will be easier. You will already know the documentation used and will probably have practised performing an admission as a student.
- If this is not your training hospital, the documentation is likely to be very different. Ask your mentor to go through the documents required (the admission sheet, discharge planner, care plans, etc.).
- Documentation is very important and will ensure that your patient receives the best care. It will allow for a smooth discharge and referrals.
- The more admissions you do, the quicker you will become. The first few will take you quite a long time, but as you become used to the sort of questions you need to ask and the paperwork, this will improve.
- Look at the types of care plans that are used. Are they pre-printed or handwritten? Perhaps they are stored on the computer, or the records may be totally electronic. In this case you may need to attend an IT course.

What to do in the event of a death

- You will need to know your Trust's procedure in the event of a patient dying.
- Find out about the last offices. For example, some Trusts remove all cannulas and catheters, etc., while others leave them *in situ*. This will normally depend on the undertakers that work with the hospital.
- Is there a booklet that you can give to relatives? This is really helpful, as they will probably forget most of what you tell them. It is a good idea to read it yourself as you will probably learn a lot, and it will mean that you are supporting the information that is in the booklet.

- Find out when the relatives can collect the death certificate. This may be the next day, after a certain time. You will need to contact the Patient's Affairs department.

- What happens to the patient's property if the relative is not there to take it home? Think about what you are putting into a property bag to give to the relatives. Will they really want a soiled nightdress? Do they want spare incontinence pads? Will they want a mouldy piece of fruit? Receiving the property will be a lasting memory for that relative, and this should be undertaken with dignity for the deceased patient. Make sure that clothes are neatly folded and not merely thrown into the bag. If belongings are slightly soiled, put them in a separate bag and mark them in some way as being soiled. If there are any valuables, ensure that they are placed in the correct envelope used by the Trust. Glasses and hearing aids should be placed in a pot to protect them. Any valuables that have been stored in the safe should be signed for and placed with other valuables in the correct envelope.

- Make sure that you have access to information about different cultures and religions. This information may affect the way in which you care for the deceased patient and their relatives.

- Ensure that you talk to the other patients about the death, especially if they were sharing a bay with the deceased patient. Most of them will realise that the patient was seriously ill and may be very upset. They will need support from you. Think about how you will deal with the removal of the body from the ward area. Is it necessary to pull the curtains around each bed in the bay when the porters come to collect the body? If you have spoken to the other patients and explained what has happened, they may prefer not to have their curtains pulled. Think about how this looks to the patients – they watch while doctors and nurses do their best to save the patient's life, and then activity seems to stop. The next thing they know, the curtains are all being pulled, and when they are pulled back the bed is freshly made and the patient has disappeared. During this time no one has taken the time to talk to them about the fact that the patient has died. Perhaps it is more beneficial for the other patients to see the mortuary trolley and be sure of what is going on, rather than imagine what has happened. Of course you need to maintain confidentiality, but there is no reason why you can't be open and honest with them.

Ward philosophy of care

Find out whether your ward has a philosophy of care. If it does, this should be displayed in an area that is accessible to patients and relatives. If it does not, perhaps this is something you may want to initiate. This is very important as it gives the team a focus and states the care that will be given and the standard of that care.

Doctors' rota

- Locate the doctors' rota and ask how this works. It can be very complicated and will be different during the night and at weekends. Find out how you can know which team is 'on call' and who to bleep out of hours.
- Your Trust may operate a zoning system. This means that wards take patients from certain consultants. This system works very well, as the staff on the ward become familiar with the doctors on that team, and those doctors will be more accessible if they only have a few wards to deal with.

Nursing rota

- Ask about the procedure for requesting your off duty. For example, there may be a request book for you to ask for a certain day off, and there may be a date by which all requests have to be written in.
- Remember that compiling the off duty is very difficult, and large numbers of requests make this even harder! Try to keep them to a minimum.
- Find out the procedure for requesting annual leave. Is it via the request book, or do you have to fill in a request form or just speak to the ward manager? This will be a new concept for you. For the past few years you have been told when you will be working and when your holidays will be. You are now in control! Don't forget to take your leave. Some staff realise halfway through the year that they have not taken any leave, and then have to cram it all into six months, which can be very difficult.

Senior nurse support

This will be available in various ways and from different people.

- *Ward manager.* This person will usually be your first port of call. Go to them with any problems or issues that you are unable to resolve yourself. They would rather know as soon as possible if there is a problem before it becomes more difficult to solve. They are there to support and guide you in your development. You should be offered continual feedback on your progress, and if you are not, you should ask for it. Sometimes staff forget to tell you when you've done something well and only point out the areas that need improvement. Most Trusts have a system of appraisal, which is usually undertaken annually. This gives you the opportunity to have dedicated time with the ward manager to discuss your progress and identify any training needs.

* *Directorate manager/senior nurse/modern matron.* You will find that this person may have a different title to those listed here, but they will do the same job. They are the next line of management and will manage your manager! They will have an overview of a particular directorate (e.g. medicine or surgery), and they are responsible for ensuring that the ward managers are supported and that their wards are well staffed and productive. They will be concerned with budgets and development of the ward areas.

* *Senior nurse on call.* Out of hours there will usually be a senior nurse to cover the hospital. The advice and support of this person are invaluable. You will not be expected to take charge of the ward at present, but when you do it is very comforting to know that there is someone to turn to if you are unsure about anything. They will be able to help with staffing problems and issues regarding prescriptions, patients' relatives or any other problems that you are unable to resolve.

* *On-call manager.* This will be a member of the senior management team. They will be on call, but not usually within the hospital. The senior nurse on call will be able to contact them for advice if, for example, he/she cannot resolve a particular problem or there is a major incident.

* *Director of Nursing.* This will be the person with overall responsibility for nursing within the Trust. He/she will oversee the management of the nurses and deal with issues in conjunction with the directorate managers and ward managers. He/she will have a strategic role in ensuring that the nursing care is of a high standard, that wards are adequately staffed and that nursing is well represented both

within the Trust and in outside agencies such as the Workforce Development Confederation.

Working on the nurse 'bank' or doing extra shifts

- You may wish to supplement your salary by working extra shifts. Most Trusts have a system whereby this can be arranged. You will probably need to contact the human resources department to apply and be interviewed.
- You will then be able to inform this department of when you will be available, and they will fit you in with the shifts requested by the ward managers.
- Working extra shifts is a good way of experiencing other wards and areas of the hospital. This may give you an idea of where you would like to work in the future. You will also be able to build upon the skills you are gaining in your permanent post.
- Ensure that you do not work too many extra shifts, as this could affect your permanent job with regard to tiredness. You will need to balance the need for extra cash with the need for time off!

Electronic equipment

- Find out where to obtain equipment. For example, you may require a pump to commence an infusion. The Trust may have a central point where all equipment is stored and maintained, or each ward may have its own supply.
- You may need to attend a study day on the use of some electronic equipment. If so, ask your ward manager about this.
- Find out what to do with faulty equipment.

Important policies

All Trusts will have policies and procedures that all staff must adhere to. Find out where you can locate these policies. You do not need to know them all word for word, but you should be able to access them when required. The most important ones to look at include the following:

- how to report accidents or untoward incidents
- what to do with patients' property
- the nursing policies
- health and safety policies
- violence and aggression
- confused patients
- the complaints procedure
- reporting unsafe practice
- drug error policy
- major incident policy.

What are your personal objectives?

You may have some objectives that you feel are important over the next few weeks. These may include skills in which you feel that you have not had much experience, or objectives specific to the ward on which you are working. Use the grid overleaf to record them, and then discuss them with your mentor, who can help you to arrange them.

Short-term objectives	By when?
1	
2	
3	
4	
5	
6	
Longer-term objectives	By when?
1	
2	
3	
4	

3

Drug safety

This will be one of the areas you will be worrying about most. It may be that you have not had much experience of drug rounds during your training. You may be required to undertake assessed drug rounds. This will ensure that both you and your mentor are confident that you are competent. You will normally need to do a set number of assessed rounds, but if you still do not feel confident you must tell your mentor. It may be that you need more experience to really feel competent. You will feel very conscious of the fact that you are taking much longer than the other nurses on the ward to do your drug rounds. This is completely acceptable, and your manager would worry if you were as quick as someone who had been qualified for ten years. Because you will need to look up many of the drugs you are giving in the *British National Formulary* (*BNF*), you are bound to take longer. Don't be tempted to give a drug when you don't know what it is or its actions, just to save time. It is more important to be safe than to do your drug round quickly. If you make a drug error at this early stage, your confidence will be reduced further at a time when you already feel less confident than the experienced staff.

Your objectives

The following are examples of the types of criteria you will be required to meet.

- Look after the drug trolley. This includes making sure that you keep the trolley clean and tidy, and ensuring that if you finish a packet or bottle of tablets, you replace them ready for the next person who will be using the trolley. Ensure that you always lock the trolley when you are not near it – for example, you may have to go to the drug cupboard. If you do not lock it, a confused patient or a 'dodgy' relative may help themselves!

- Ensure that you have the correct drug chart. A patient label on the front is best (make sure that the details are correct first!). This eliminates mistakes due to poor handwriting, and you will have both the hospital number and the date of birth of the patient.

- Check the prescription, making sure that each drug is prescribed correctly. Check the date, drug, dose, signature, valid period, times to be given, when it was last given, appropriate route (e.g. if the drug was originally prescribed intravenously, whether it still needs to be administered via this route), and lastly whether the drug interacts with any others on the chart.

- Check the chart for indications of allergies. These should also be indicated by a different-coloured wrist band (usually red). Most importantly, always check with the patient, as the doctor may not have identified an allergy.

- You *must not* give any drug unless you know what it is. If you ignore this advice and the patient is prescribed another drug, for example, that has the same action, they may become seriously ill. You would not have a leg to stand on if you were asked 'Why did you give the drug when the patient is on another drug that does the same thing?' (e.g. a beta-blocker). If you answer 'I didn't know it was a beta-blocker,' you will be asked 'Why did you give the drug if you didn't know what it was?'. The fact that the doctor had prescribed it is no defence. As a registered nurse you must know what drugs you are administering. This will mean that at first you will be much slower than other nurses who have been qualified for some time. This does not matter – it is more important to be safe than fast. Your colleagues will be anticipating that you may be slower than them, and if you are not they will be worried! Ensure you have a copy of the *BNF* on the trolley, and use it as much as you need to. Remember that you can also ask the other staff nurses if you are unsure about anything.

- Always check the container for the name of the drug, the dose and the expiry date. Don't forget to check the strip if the container is a box, as someone may have put the wrong strip into the wrong box.

- You must always question a prescription if you think there is something wrong with it. You may think that the dose is unusual (a good tip is that if the dose prescribed means that you are dispensing five tablets, for example, it may be wrong – most tablets will match the dose prescribed or be half or a third of the dose, but not usually more than this). You may be unable to read the doctor's handwriting – a very common problem. Don't guess what it says, but ask the doctor to rewrite it. They may not be very happy about this, but it is not worth risking your registration for the sake of upsetting a doctor. In any case, most will not mind.

- Check your patient's vital signs before you give them their drugs, especially if they are taking beta-blockers, vasodilators, digitalis, diuretics or anti-hypertensives. This may mean doing your patient's observations before the drug round if there is no one else to do them for you. If you give a dose of an antihypertensive and the patient is already hypotensive, you may cause them to become seriously ill. Once you have given the tablet, you can't take it back!

- Question the prescription if you think that the drug may cause problems for your patient. For example, they may be prescribed analgesia that can cause disorientation or drowsiness. The patient may be more drowsy or confused that morning, so giving the drug may make the situation worse. You must not give drugs 'blindly' – you are a *thinking* nurse.

- Ensure that you are confident about giving drugs via a variety of routes. As a student you may not have practised giving drugs via a nasogastric tube very much. Ask a more senior member of staff to check that you are doing it correctly. Know your limitations.

- When you have dispensed the tablets into a pot, take them to the patient. Always check the name band with the drug card, even if you know the patient really well. It is easy to become distracted and you may inadvertently go to the wrong patient.

- You must always ensure that the patient has taken the drugs that you have given them. A friend of mine was doing a drug round when she was newly qualified, and she left a pot of tablets on the table of her patient and went on to the next patient. Unfortunately, the healthcare assistant came along behind her and put the table in front of another patient, who then took the tablets believing that they were for him. The patient may also drop the tablets or lose one of them. You may not be able to work out what has been lost if the tablets look similar.

- Ensure that you sign the drug chart correctly. If you forget to sign it, the next person doing the drugs for that patient may think they have missed that drug and give it again. If you omit a drug for any reason, make sure that you record this on the chart in the designated place. Do not just put a cross in the box, as the next nurse will not know if it was a doctor or a nurse who crossed it off or why it wasn't given. You may forget to pass on to your colleague the fact that you have missed something out and why. Good documentation is one of the keys to safety.

- As a qualified nurse, you are fully accountable for the drugs that you administer. Even if the doctor has prescribed a drug incorrectly, you are expected to know this and not give the drug. If you are not sure, ask the doctor to clarify the dose/drug. If you are still not happy with the response, check with a more senior doctor or the nurse in charge. You can also ask the pharmacist or senior nurse on call. There will always be someone to ask, so don't be pressurised into giving something that you think is wrong. Some Trusts will have a procedure for disagreement over a prescription. If so, you must follow this.
- Ensure that drugs are stored according to hospital policy.
- Make sure that you know what to do if your patient experiences anaphylactic shock and what the signs are. Some drugs may cause these symptoms in a small number of patients. Less severe reactions such as rashes are more common. Any reaction should be discussed with the patient's doctor and documented before the next dose is administered.
- Ask a member of the team to advise you of the most common drugs that are used on the ward. You can then ensure that you know the actions, side-effects, contraindications and dosages for these. You will not be expected to know every drug, but if you don't you would be expected to find out the information.
- Find out how to order drugs if necessary and how the stock is maintained. How can you obtain drugs when the pharmacy is closed out of hours? Is there an emergency drug cupboard? Is there a pharmacist on call?
- If you find that there is no stock on the ward of a particular drug that you require, it is important that you obtain and administer that drug as soon as possible. Ensure that you record on the drug card that there is 'no stock' – do not just write NS (no stock) in the box, as this could look like

someone's initials. Order the required drug from the pharmacy and administer it as soon as it arrives on the ward. Do not leave it until the next drug round, or even the next day, if it is a once-a-day drug! This may sound obvious, but some nurses will write 'no stock' in the box and then take no action to obtain the drug or administer it when it arrives. This may be seen as negligent and/or an omission of care, especially if the patient's condition deteriorates as a result.

- Find out about the Take Home Drugs service and how this is organised. Some hospitals reuse the drugs that patients have brought into hospital and others don't. Find out how long a supply is given so that you can advise your patient regarding a repeat prescription when they get home. What happens to the discharge letter? Does it get sent automatically from the pharmacy to the GP or do you need to do this? Does the patient receive a copy? Think about the advice you will need to give regarding the medications. For example, the patient may be going home on anticoagulants, so will need advice about what to do if bleeding occurs and how to arrange follow-up appointments, etc.

- Ask about the policy regarding controlled drugs. Make sure that you know how your hospital expects you to record what you have given, who should check them and how they should be administered. Where are they stored and how do you access them?

- Ensure that you have a copy of the Nursing and Midwifery Council (NMC) *Guidelines for the Administration of Medicines* (2002). Adhere to this at all times and both you and your patients will be safe.

Intravenous infusions

As a student nurse you may not have been allowed to perform this skill fully. Consequently, many newly qualified nurses worry about practising setting up, commencing and maintaining infusions correctly.

Cannula care

This is a very important aspect of intravenous therapy. Without a patent cannula, you will not be able to infuse the prescribed fluids. The cannula must be inspected daily and appropriate action taken if it is not patent.

Check the following.

- Is the dressing secure and clean? If not, change it. This will be an infection risk if it is left dirty and bloodstained. If it is not secure, the cannula may be displaced accidentally.
- Are there any signs of infection or irritation? Look at the skin surrounding the entry site and check for redness, pain, swelling and/or exudate. Any redness may 'track' upwards following the vein. If you suspect that the cannula may be displaced or infected, ask a colleague who has gained their IV drug administration certificate to check the patency by attempting to flush the cannula. Remove the cannula if infection or displacement is suspected, and ensure that a new cannula is inserted as soon as possible.
- Do they still require the cannula? If it is not being used for the administration of fluids or drugs and does not need to be there prophylactically (e.g. for a patient who is likely to bleed), it should be removed as it will be an infection risk. It will be unlikely to be patent if it has not been used for several days.

Infusion safety

The procedure is as follows.

1 Check that the prescription is valid.
2 Check the correct fluids with another qualified nurse (check your policy).
3 Ensure that you have the correct giving set. If the fluids are to be infused via a pump, you will need a specific set.
4 If you are infusing the fluids via a pump, ensure that you have attended the appropriate course (some Trusts require this).
5 Explain to your patient what you are doing and why.
6 Check the prescription against the patient's ID band.
7 Prime the giving set, ensuring that there are no air bubbles.
8 Attach it to the cannula. This may require flushing by a qualified colleague if it has not been used for a few hours.
9 Calculate the correct drip rate according to the prescription. Think about your patient's condition. For example, if they have known congestive cardiac failure and the prescription states that the infusion should run over 2 hours, this will need to be questioned with the prescribing doctor.
10 Open the roller clamp and set the drip rate.
11 Ensure that the patient is comfortable.
12 Document the infusion using a fluid chart, and sign the prescription sheet.
13 Ensure that you have enough fluids prescribed for the next 24 hours.

4

The next two to six weeks

You are probably no longer supernumerary, and it's time to get really stuck in! Now is the time when you will get your own group of patients to care for without working alongside another staff nurse. Scary – or is it? You've settled in and know the routine, and you should always be working with someone more senior than yourself. So don't worry about it, and enjoy having your 'own' patients and putting all you have learned into practice. Over the next few weeks you will need to learn about the following.

When to contact doctors

This is a very difficult area, especially when you are newly qualified. You will want to contact them as soon as you are worried about a patient or have a question about their treatment.

Try to resist the temptation to bleep them, and instead ask a more senior nurse what they think you should do. Remember that you may be interrupting an important discussion with a relative, for example, or the doctor may be performing a clinical procedure. However, they do not mind if you bleep them about reasonable problems.

Speak to the nurse in charge, as they may be able to answer your question. They may also know that another nurse has bleeped the doctor and he/she is coming up to the ward shortly. It may be that your query can wait until they arrive on the ward.

The nurse in charge may advise you to discuss your question with someone other than that particular doctor, perhaps the pharmacist.

He/she may confirm that you do need to bleep the doctor, but that you should have certain information to hand. For example, if you are worried about the patient's condition, you will need to know their vital signs, fluid balance, oxygen saturations, blood sugar levels and level of responsiveness.

Preparation for theatre/investigations

The principles are always the same, whether you are preparing a patient for theatre or an invasive investigation. So long as you follow these basic guidelines, the patient and you will be safe.

- Check that the patient has given adequate consent. Have they signed the consent form? Do they understand what the doctor has said to them? Do they understand what their options are?
- Check that the patient is wearing an identity band. This should state the patient's name, hospital number and date of birth. These details must correspond exactly to the notes and the X-rays. If the patient has an allergy, this should also be indicated – usually with a separate red band.
- If the operation requires the site to be marked, check that this has been done and that it corresponds with the notes. For example, if the notes say 'left below-knee amputation', ensure that the doctor has marked the left leg! This may sound obvious, but believe it or not mistakes such as this are actually made.

- Make sure that the patient has been allowed nil by mouth for the required period of time. This time may vary depending on the type of operation or investigation. If they have not fasted for some reason, you must inform the doctor, as the procedure may have to be postponed due to the risk of vomiting and aspiration. Some procedures may only require the patient to be allowed clear fluids. There will usually be a resource file on the ward for you to find this information.

- Ensure that you record a set of 'baseline' observations prior to the operation/procedure. This will be of benefit to the theatre staff when they are recording the patient's vital signs peri- and post-operatively, as they will be able to compare them to see if, for example, hypertension is usual for that patient.

- Ask the patient whether they have any loose teeth or crowns. The anaesthetist will need to know this so that they can avoid that area of the mouth when intubating. Otherwise the patient may lose the tooth or crown or may even aspirate it.

- Find out about prosthetics or metal plates, as these may affect X-rays or diathermy. The surgeon will also want this information if they are operating on that part of the body – they will not want any surprises!

- If the patient is diabetic, ensure that this is well catered for pre-operatively. If they are insulin controlled, they will probably require intravenous sliding-scale insulin and IV fluids. If not, they will require close monitoring of their blood glucose levels and perhaps some IV fluids. You should record their blood glucose levels before the procedure, again to provide a set of baseline data.

- Make sure that the patient is not wearing any make-up or nail varnish, so that their skin colour can be seen during the procedure. Nail varnish may also affect the oxygen saturation probe so that it cannot read the level. Don't assume that this only applies to female patients! Men and boys have often been found to be wearing either nail varnish or make-up (sometimes both!).

- Make sure that all jewellery and hair clips are removed. Check your Trust's policy with regard to wedding rings – you may be able to tape them, as most patients do not want to remove them. As piercings are becoming more common, you will need to find out the Trust policy with regard to their removal.
- Find out whether the patient wears contact lenses, as they will need to be removed prior to the procedure. Hearing aids will also need to be removed, and you must ensure that you inform the theatre staff so that they are aware that the patient may not be able to hear them.
- Ensure that you have completed the checklist required and that all of the necessary documentation goes to theatre with the patient. You will be required to hand over this information to the nurse in theatre.

Post-operative care

Again the principles will be the same regardless of the operation or procedure that the patient has undergone.

- When you go to the recovery area you must ensure:
  - that the patient is conscious. They may be drowsy, but they should be responsive and able to maintain their own airway. If they are not, you must not accept them back into your care, but insist that they remain in the recovery area until it is safe to transfer them back to the ward. This may be inconvenient for the staff in Recovery, but remember that the patient's safety is more important. The staff will then contact the ward when the patient is ready

- that you have read the peri-operative notes and the post-operative instructions. You need to know what has already been done and what needs to be done when the patient is back on the ward
- that you inspect the wound site. There may be some blood on the dressing, but the wound should not be actively bleeding. If it is, you must insist that the surgeon inspects the wound prior to taking the patient from the recovery area
- that you have looked at the recorded observations and discussed any problems with the recovery nurse
- that you have discussed any pain relief given while the patient was in theatre and recovery, as this is not always obvious when you are looking at the notes. You do not want to get back to the ward and give the same drug that they may have recently received while in theatre
- that you discuss any wound drains and that they are not already full – this may indicate excessive bleeding. Again you will need to check this with the surgeon
- that you discuss any problems that have occurred, and the outcome.

- When you return to the ward:
  - ensure that you perform regular observations on your patient. This will usually be every 30 minutes for the first 2 hours, and thereafter will depend on the patient's condition, but you will need to check the Trust policy
  - document in the nursing notes what has happened and the post-operative instructions. It is important to document any untoward incidents that may have occurred in theatre or recovery
  - talk to your patient about what has happened and what they can expect over the next few hours and days. This will aid their recovery. Discuss pain relief and how often they can receive it. If they have a patient-controlled analgesia

(PCA) pump *in situ*, make sure that they understand how to use it. Ensure that you perform regular checks with regard to the PCA. How often you need to do this will depend on your Trust policy. It is very important that these checks are made to ensure the patient's safety while they are receiving these powerful drugs. Report any abnormal observations at once to the nurse/doctor in charge

– check the wound site when you check the vital signs for excessive bleeding or opening of the wound, and report any unusual findings immediately to the doctor. If this does occur you will need to apply pressure to the wound until assistance arrives. Occasionally the patient may have to return to theatre to have a drain inserted or the wound resutured

– if the relatives want to be informed as soon as the patient is back on the ward, remember to contact them. They may be extremely anxious and waiting on the end of the phone for your call and reassurance that their loved one is OK

– provide food and drink as soon as the patient is allowed to eat and drink. The time will vary depending on the operation/procedure performed. Most patients will be desperate for a cup of tea!

Nasogastric (NG) tubes

Your patient may well require a nasogastric tube during their hospital stay, whether on a surgical or medical ward. It is important to know how to insert one correctly and care for it once it is *in situ*. This may be a skill you did not have the opportunity to master as a student, as some universities do not allow their students to practise this, especially if the Trusts to which they send students consider this to be an extended role that requires further training. Now is the time to make sure that you get as much practice as possible. If this is something you have never done, ask if you can watch the first time and then practise under the supervision of an experienced staff nurse.

If the Trust you are working in requires extra training, ensure that you access this as soon as possible. Before you attempt to pass a tube, always check that there are no contraindicating factors, such as stomach cancer or recent surgery on any part of the digestive tract.

There are two types of NG tube:

1 a fine-bore tube which contains a metal introducer. This is used in cases where the tube is likely to be *in situ* for a long period of time (e.g. when parenteral feeding is required). It must be X-rayed once *in situ* to check its position, as it is so fine that it could pass into the lungs

2 a Ryles tube, which has a larger lumen and no introducer. This is used post-operatively (e.g. for a short period of time when a patient has an obstruction and fluid needs to be drained from the stomach). Its position can be checked using a stethoscope and/or litmus paper.

The procedure for passing an NG tube can be summarised as follows.

1 Explain to the patient exactly what you are about to do and why, and obtain their consent. If they have had this proce-dure done before, they are likely to be extremely anxious, as it can be a very unpleasant and painful experience.

2 Obtain the necessary equipment:
   * NG tube – e.g. Ryles tube (without an introducer) or fine bore depending on the purpose of the tube
   * water-based lubricating jelly

- litmus paper
- syringe – 10 ml
- stethoscope
- adhesive tape – check that the patient does not have an allergy to this
- safety pin
- glass of water
- gloves.

3   Measure the required length of tube, so that you know approximately how much needs to be passed. You can measure this by taking the tube and holding one end to the patient's ear lobe, then guiding it to the tip of their nose and down to the sternal notch. This will give you the approximate length. Make a note of where this is on the tube. Most tubes will have a series of marks along their length.

4   Put on a pair of gloves (they do not need to be sterile).

5   Place a small amount of jelly on the end of the tube.

6   Explain to your patient again what you are going to do. Ask them to put their chin on their chest, as this will help to close off the airway, thus reducing the risk of the tube passing into the trachea.

7   If your patient is able to drink, give them a glass of water and ask them to swallow some when you ask them to. If they cannot drink, ask them to try to swallow, again when you ask them to. This helps to pass the tube down.

8   Place the tip of the tube into either nostril, avoiding using a nostril in which any trauma is present.

9   Commence passing the tube, asking the patient to swallow, with water if possible. Try to pass the tube at a continuous rate, avoiding a large number of stops and starts, as this will prolong the experience for the patient. However, if the patient starts to cough violently or becomes cyanosed, you must stop immediately, as this

may be an indication that the tube is in the trachea. Once you stop, the patient may recover and you may be able to continue.

Sometimes the patient will automatically cough as the tube is passed through the back of the throat. If you are concerned that it is in the trachea, remove the tube immediately. If you are happy to continue, pass the tube until the mark that you measured beforehand is reached.

10   Tape the tube on to the nose.

11   If a fine-bore tube is passed, you will need to send the patient to X-ray to check the position once the doctor has signed the X-ray form. This must then be checked by the doctor before feeding is commenced. Document in the patient's notes the name of the doctor who checked the X-ray and what their conclusion was. Practise looking at the X-rays yourself so that you can reassure yourself that you know the tube is in the right place before feeding the patient. Remember that some junior doctors may have seen fewer of these X-rays than you. It is possible to check the position using air, but this can be difficult due to the introducer. Once the position has been confirmed, remove the guide-wire.

12   If you are using a Ryles tube, you can check the position in two ways. First, you can listen to the stomach using a stethoscope and insert 10 ml of air into the end of the tube. If the tube is in the stomach you will hear a gurgling sound. If you do not hear anything, try using the litmus method. This involves withdrawing a small amount of gastric fluid from the tube and using litmus paper to check the pH. If the paper turns red, this indicates acid and the tube is in the stomach. Personally I like to do both of these to double check. This may not be possible if the patient has been nil by mouth for some time, as there may be nothing in the stomach to aspirate.

13 Whenever you are restarting a feed or giving medications via the tube, always recheck the position in case the patient has pulled the tube out of position.

14 Aftercare involves ensuring that the patient is comfortable and that the tube is not causing trauma to the nasal passages. Most patients find these tubes uncomfortable and may complain of a sore throat, especially with Ryles tubes (due to their having a larger lumen). Place a piece of tape around the tube and pin it to the patient's clothing to prevent them accidentally catching the tube and pulling it out.

Percutaneous endoscopically guided gastrostomy (PEG) tubes

PEG tubes are inserted when a patient requires long-term nutritional support. They are convenient and discrete for patients who may need to go home with supplemental feeding.

PEG tubes are inserted surgically, and therefore require the pre-operative checks discussed earlier in this chapter.

Post-operative care involves recording the patient's vital signs and observing for signs of internal bleeding. Observe the site for signs of swelling, excoriation and irritation. Note on the measuring device on the tube where it enters the skin. This will reassure you that the tube has not been misplaced when you come to check it daily. The tube should be cleaned aseptically daily using 0.9% sterile sodium chloride and gauze, and inspected for signs of infection or irritation. There is no need to dress the tube following removal of the post-procedural dressing, unless the wound is leaking or exuding fluid.

Advise the patient not to use creams or talcum powder around the site, to prevent infection or irritation. Once the patient is home, they can use regular soap and water.

Enteral feeding

Enteral feeding occurs via an NG or PEG tube, and will be considered for patients who are unable to meet their nutritional requirements through their oral intake. This may be due to trauma to the gastrointestinal tract (e.g. oesophageal surgery), neurological disorders (e.g. a cerebrovascular accident), psychological disorders (e.g. anorexia nervosa), obstruction of the gastrointestinal tract (e.g. cancer of the oesophagus) or a non-functioning gastrointestinal tract (e.g. bowel obstruction).

The feeding regime and type of feed will be determined by the dietitian. Feeding will be commenced slowly and built up gradually to ensure that the gastrointestinal tract does not react to the feed. The latter sometimes causes loose stools and nausea if commenced too quickly. The regime and amount of feed will depend on whether the patient can supplement this with any oral intake. The regime may also include water, especially at the beginning, to ensure that enough fluid is taken. Often the aim will be to give the regime overnight. This should always be the case if possible, so that during the day the patient is 'free' for their rehabilitation (e.g. if the patient has had a cerebrovascular accident). This also means that if the patient is going home with the NG or PEG tube, they will be able to do other things during the day, rather than being attached to the feeding pump. The patient will need to be taught how to maintain the feeding tube, etc. if they are to return home with it.

Urinary catheterisation

Most Trusts require staff nurses to attend a course on re-catheterisation of male patients, due to potential problems with regard to the prostate. If this is the case, this skill will need to be assessed and updated yearly.

Female catheterisation is a skill in which many student nurses do not feel they have had enough practice during their training. Consequently, as newly qualified nurses they are very anxious about this procedure. This is compounded by the fact that it is a procedure that most patients find extremely embarrassing and it can be quite uncomfortable. So obviously you will want to get it right! If you have not had much experience, the earlier you are able to consolidate this skill the better. Ask a more experienced nurse to come with you and assist you the first couple of times. They will be able to guide you if you experience any difficulties.

You will need the following equipment:

- clean trolley
- catheter (the size will depend on the type of drainage required – the more likely the urine is to contain clots, the larger the lumen required. You may also need to consider the size of any previous catheter); take two catheters with you
- 0.9% sterile sodium chloride
- 10-ml sterile syringe
- sterile water for injections (10 ml)
- sterile gloves
- anaesthetic gel
- catheter bag and stand
- sterile catheter/dressing pack
- specimen pot if a specimen is required.

The procedure is as follows.

1   Explain to the patient what you are intending to do and why. Obtain their verbal consent.
2   Maintain the patient's privacy and dignity by ensuring

that colleagues do not disturb you and that the curtains are securely closed.

3   Attempt to relax the patient, as they will be embarrassed and anxious. Chat to them.

4   Assist the patient into a position where they have their heels as close to their buttocks as possible, and ask them to let their legs fall apart. Once they have done this, cover them with a sheet until you are ready. An assistant can help the patient to stay in this position, especially if they are elderly and not very flexible!

5   Apply anaesthetic gel to the urethral opening.

6   Prepare the trolley so that everything is easily to hand.

7   Wash your hands.

8   Using aseptic technique, put on your gloves.

9   Empty the saline into the pot provided within the catheter/dressing pack.

10   Draw up 10 ml of saline water into the syringe.

11   Using one hand only, clean the genital area with the saline and gauze, using each piece of gauze for one wipe only. Use your 'clean' hand to wet the gauze and then pass it to your 'dirty' hand to wipe. Once you are satisfied that the area is clean you can proceed.

12   Undo the sheath covering the catheter at the tip end and peel back for approximately 6 or 7 cm.

13   Identify the urethral opening and insert the tip of the catheter into the urethra. Using gentle pressure, insert the tube into the urethra until you can see urine appearing at the open end of the tube. This is the reason for leaving the plastic sheath on the catheter – it will catch the urine and prevent it from spilling out on to the bed.

14   Place the open end into the plastic tray in your pack and remove the plastic sheath.

15   Insert 10 ml of sterile water into the port of the catheter to inflate the balloon.

16   Gently pull the catheter out until you feel resistance – this means that the balloon is sitting in the entrance of the bladder in the correct position.

17   Attach the catheter bag and ensure that the bag is secured to a stand and not left in the bed or on the floor!

18   Ensure that the patient is comfortable, and if you did spill any urine on the sheet make certain that this is replaced. Inform the patient that the catheter will be emptied regularly and that they should drink plenty of water (unless they are fluid restricted) in order to prevent urinary tract infections and to keep the tube patent. They should be advised that catheter care will be given twice daily or more often if required, and if they are able the patient can be taught how to do this, especially if they will be discharged with the catheter *in situ*.

19   Observe whether any immediate residual volume is passed. If it is, record the amount and inform the doctors that there was a residual amount of urine, as this may indicate that the patient's bladder was in retention.

The genital area should be washed twice daily with soap and water. A disposable cloth should be used, and when cleaning around the entry site of the catheter the cloth should be discarded after each wipe and a new one used. The area should be dried thoroughly and talcum powder should not be used, as this can irritate the genital area and may cause infection. The contents of the tube and catheter bag should be inspected for signs of infection (debris, offensive odour and cloudiness). If infection is suspected, a specimen should be taken and should be sent to the microbiology department for microbiology, culture and sensitivity (MC&S). If the urine appears dark, this may indicate that the patient is dehydrated, and they should be encouraged to drink at least one and a half litres of water daily (unless they are fluid restricted).

The catheter bag should be kept below the level of the patient's waist to prevent urine flowing back up the tube and into the bladder, thereby increasing the risk of infection.

Blood transfusion

It is very important that you find out the policy within your Trust for the transfusion of blood products. Blood transfusion errors are potentially fatal, so you must ensure that you are safe and knowledgeable with regard to this practice.

Whatever the policy, the principles will be the same.

- The blood product should be checked at the patient's bedside for name, date of birth, hospital number, blood group, expiry date, valid prescription and blood identification number. These details must be checked with the patient, the ID band and the notes, by two qualified nurses. As a student you may not have had the opportunity to check the blood, depending on your university and Trust policy. There is no reason why a student nurse cannot observe and practise checking as a third 'checker'. If any discrepancy is identified when checking the blood, *do not start the transfusion*. Always ask for advice and report any problems. Occasionally patients are able to receive blood from blood groups other than their own, but you must always check with the pathology department if the blood you receive is not the patient's known blood group.
- If the patient is prescribed any diuretics, ensure that these are given at the same time as the blood. This is to prevent the patient from becoming fluid overloaded. Diuretics will not be prescribed for all patients, but usually for those with cardiac failure. If you feel that your patient should have diuretics prescribed, but they do not, check with the

doctor, as they may have been overlooked.

- The patient's vital signs (blood pressure, respiratory rate, pulse rate and temperature) must be recorded according to Trust policy. The frequency will usually be as follows:
  - baseline observations before the transfusion is commenced
  - observation of vital signs every 5 minutes for the first 15 minutes
  - thereafter, hourly observations throughout the transfusion
  - all observations must be documented
  - any change from the baseline observations must be reported to the doctor and the transfusion stopped until the patient has been seen by the doctor.
- Document in the medical notes the units of blood transfused. Sometimes this is done by attaching the label from the bag of blood to the appropriate page of the notes.
- Document the transfusion in the nursing notes, noting any issues that have arisen.
- Observe the patient for signs of adverse reactions such as a rash or flushing. Ask them to inform you if they experience any symptoms such as headache, breathlessness or nausea.
- Ensure that the blood is transfused over the prescribed period of time. Always check with the doctor if you think the time period may be too long or too short. For example, the patient may have cardiac failure, and if the blood is prescribed to be transfused over 2 hours, they may experience shortness of breath indicating fluid overload.
- Your patient may be prescribed more than one unit of blood, in which case the same procedure must be followed for each separate bag. If the transfusion is not urgent, check with the doctor whether the transfusion warrants disruption to your patient's sleep. In some Trusts it is policy not

to transfuse overnight except in an emergency. This decreases the risk to patient safety.
- Following the completion of the transfusion, the cannula must be cleared of blood by flushing the line with saline. You will need to ask a senior colleague to do this, as this procedure requires further IV training. This will ensure that the cannula remains patent and does not become blocked with clotted blood.

If you have a transfusion nurse specialist working within your Trust, it will be beneficial for you to arrange to spend some time with them. They will be able to update you on recent developments and the Trust policies.

Referrals

Make sure that you can refer appropriately to the following:

- discharge nurse
- physiotherapist
- occupational therapist
- speech therapist
- dietitians
- social services
- clinical nurse specialists
- case managers
- district nurse
- nurse consultants.

Find out who nurses can refer to and which disciplines require a medical referral. You may need to ensure that this is documented in the patient's notes, or it may be necessary to complete a referral form.

Clinical supervision and reflection

Clinical supervision is an important part of developing as a competent practitioner. You will experience many situations over the course of your career. As a newly qualified nurse, these situations may appear more complicated than you will find them in a few years' time! However, clinical supervision will be every bit as necessary in 10 years' time as it is now. The nursing profession is constantly changing and developing, and therefore you should never feel as if you know everything there is to know. Supervision is concerned with helping you to make sense of situations that you have experienced. Your supervisor may be someone you currently work with, or someone from a different ward or department. Some Trusts have a list of clinical supervisors, and you may be free to choose your own, while other Trusts may allocate a supervisor to you. If your Trust does not offer formal supervision, you may want to ask someone with whom you get on well to meet with you regularly to discuss any issues.

Clinical supervision may be formal or informal, and may take place within a group or individually.

With the help of your supervisor, you will be able to explore issues and feelings that you may have experienced. This will enable you to develop and improve your practice and the care that you provide for your patients. Supervision is important following a stressful situation, such as an emergency. For example, you may feel that you did not react very well and perhaps you panicked – a common reaction in a newly qualified nurse. If you do not discuss this, you may find that the next time you act in the same way. However, if you have the opportunity to discuss what happened and explore what you did that was helpful and what you did that was not, you can improve your practice next time you are in the same situation. Your supervisor can reassure you and offer constructive criticism.

You may find that you have no particular issues to discuss. You may want to talk generally about your progress and what you are planning to do in the future. Your supervisor can assist you in planning which courses or experiences you may need to consider in order to develop your practice.

Reflective practice also involves putting your experiences down on paper. This is an important part of both your portfolio and your development. Once you have the chance to write something down and use a structured reflective approach, you will find that you can think about the situation more clearly.

What should I do if I make a mistake?

As in all professions that involve human workers, there will be an accepted degree of risk of human error. This must be acknowledged, and a 'no-blame culture' should be encouraged if staff are to feel supported should they make a mistake. If staff are to learn from their mistakes, each mistake must be reported and the nurse supported by discussing what went wrong and why, and what they would do differently in the future.

- The first thing you must do is to tell a senior member of staff.
- The Trust policy may state that the incident must be formally reported, and if so, this must be done as soon as possible. This will probably involve filling in an incident form. The reason for doing this is so that the hospital management team can identify trends and patterns of incidents and, if necessary, investigate them further. For example, if nurses on a particular ward repeatedly make drug errors and claim on the incident form that this is due

to lack of trained staff, the senior nurse must investigate this situation. The ward may fill out many forms involving back injuries to staff, which may be due to inadequate training and/or equipment. Again this situation must be investigated and an action plan initiated.

- If the incident involves drugs, the doctor must be informed and remedial action taken. Often no action will be required. For example, if antibiotics have been given by mistake, most patients will show no adverse effects. You may be asked to observe the patient for signs of a rash or other reactions if they are known to be allergic to these drugs. However, sometimes the patient may require close observation of their vital signs (e.g. if they are given the wrong dose of digitalis or a beta-blocker). In severe cases the patient may require transfer to a more acute area (e.g. coronary care) where counter-reactive drugs can be administered.

- Ensure that you inform your patient if you have made a mistake. It is their right to know. Most patients will react well to your honesty and accept the fact that this can happen.

- You must document in the nursing notes what has happened and the action that was taken.

- You must never worry about admitting to a mistake. It is much better to admit it at the time, rather than hope that no one notices and be found out later. That would be looked upon very seriously and disciplinary action might be taken. Unless you have been negligent or acted outside your limitations, you will not be reprimanded.

- Remember that to make a mistake is part of being human. However, making the same mistake again means that you have not learned from your mistake!

- Risk management is all about recognising the risks involved in a procedure and reducing them. This is done by using policies and procedures. If you adhere to these you will be less likely to make a mistake.

Professionalism

What does *professionalism* mean?

[It refers to] A person who engages in an activity with great competence.
(*The New Collins Dictionary and Thesaurus* 1988)

This means being consistent in your manner and actions, always being professional and ensuring that the standards of the nursing profession are always upheld.

There are many different aspects involved in professionalism.

- *The way we appear to the patients.* Wear your uniform with pride and according to the Trust's policy. Make sure that your uniform is always clean and well fitting. No jewellery should be worn, and hair should be tied back if it is below the collar line. Well-fitting, flat shoes should be worn, and no optional accessories (e.g. a stethoscope around your neck!).
- *The way we communicate with others.* Think about what you say and to whom. The patients probably don't want to know what you were doing last night! It is not professional to discuss your private life in front of patients and other staff. The staff room is the place for this type of conversation. Think about your body language. Try to be approachable to other members of the team. If you disagree with another member of the team, discuss the issue in a calm and mature way and debate rather than argue. If you find yourself in a volatile situation, move the conversation to a private area.

- *Outside work.* Although you are not on duty, remember that you are still representing the nursing profession. For example, it is not acceptable for you to wear your uniform to go to the pub after work. An identifiable nurse drinking and smoking is not the impression we should be giving to the public – it is hypocritical. Remember also that we must maintain confidentiality. Even though you may not mention a name, the person to whom you are talking may know the patient or member of staff and be able to identify who you are talking about. This would be a serious disciplinary matter if the person's confidentiality was to be breached. Think about the way you talk to others who are not nurses. We tend to have a dark sense of humour that may not be appreciated by someone outside the profession.

5

'The six-month tears'

When I first started this job, my boss, Ruth, said to me – 'Watch out for the six-month tears!' At the time I didn't really know what she meant, but now I do!

Almost all newly qualified nurses go through this stage. It may be straight away or it may be six months after qualification. They suddenly realise that they don't know enough. They panic and think they are the only person to feel like this. The reality is that most nurses feel this way when they first qualify.

This stage is usually triggered by a critical situation. The nurse may be looking after a patient who suddenly becomes very unwell. They then realise that they don't know what to do.

You need to remember that this will probably happen to you at some stage. If you are prepared for feeling like this, it will not seem so bad. Of course, it may not happen to you at all, but the vast majority of newly qualified nurses experience this feeling of being 'out of their depth'.

In order to reduce the effects of this transition period, take every opportunity to learn from those around you. During the first six months, take the time to identify any gaps in your knowledge and make every effort to fill them. Those around you will be expecting you to have lots of questions and to be feeling under-confident.

You will find that there are various ways to 'fill' these knowledge gaps:

- talking to your mentor
- clinical supervision
- working alongside more senior nurses/practice development and specialist nurses
- discussing your patients with the multi-disciplinary team and learning from their expertise.

Attending study days and courses

The following are courses that you may wish to consider during your first six months to a year post qualification:

- risk management and accountability
- venepuncture
- cannulation
- NVQ assessor
- IV drug administration
- pumps and epidurals
- high-dependency course
- ALERT/emergency situation course.

Of course, these courses will have different titles depending on which Trust you work for, but most Trusts will offer training along these lines. You will need to discuss with your mentor and/or ward manager which courses are most suitable for the area in which you are working. They may already have some continuing professional development (CPD) arranged or planned for you.

There will also be mandatory study for you to undertake on induction to the Trust. This will probably include the following:

- fire training
- moving and handling

- resuscitation
- customer care
- health and safety
- control of substances hazardous to health (COSHH)
- transfusion training
- infection control.

Ensure that you are aware of the procedure for applying for courses within your Trust. You will usually need to complete an application form, and this may need to be signed by your ward manager. Some courses will be 'in-house' and therefore free to Trust staff, while others may be offered by the local university and there may be a funding implication. Usually you can apply for part funding for these courses from the Trust. Study time is normally negotiable, depending on the relevance of the course to your area of work.

Important NMC publications

You must ensure that you have read and understand the following NMC publications:

- *Scope of Professional Practice*
- *Code of Conduct*
- *Administration of Medicines*
- *Portfolio Building and PREP*
- *Guidelines for Records and Record Keeping.*

These are the standards against which you will be measured, so it is essential that you adhere to them at all times.

Accountability

Although this has been mentioned many times already, it is so important that it deserves its own 'bit'.

You are now accountable for *everything* that you do within your role as a staff nurse. You must be sure that you can justify your actions at all times.

You are also accountable for the actions of others to whom you delegate. This means that if you delegate a task to a member of staff who is not competent and they perform the task wrongly, you are accountable for the harm caused to the patient. The member of staff is *responsible* for their actions, but you remain *accountable*.

You will also be held accountable for carrying out doctors' orders that are wrong. For example, you may give an incorrectly prescribed drug. Although the doctor is accountable for prescribing it wrongly, you will also be held accountable for administering it, as you must be sure of all drugs, dosages, actions, contraindications and side-effects of the drugs that you give to patients. In the same way, if you perform incorrectly a procedure that a doctor has asked you to do, you will be accountable. This is because you must be aware of your limitations and not carry out any procedure unless you are appropriately trained to do so. Even if you have received the recommended training, you may not have performed the skill for a period of time and are therefore not practised at the task, and thus not competent. Again, you will be held accountable if you perform the task incorrectly.

Once you start taking charge of the ward, the same principles will apply when you delegate to junior staff nurses.

6

Your first year

This is the beginning of your whole career, and now is the time to start as you mean to go on. Make sure that you are competent and efficient now and these skills will ensure that you have an enjoyable and fruitful career. During this year you will learn more than at any other time. Try to make the best of all situations, even if they don't seem very positive at the time – you can learn something from every experience. You are surrounded by knowledgeable and supportive people, so draw on this knowledge and experience from all members of the team.

During this year you will need to gain a working knowledge of, and become competent in, the following areas.

Prioritising acute care

To begin with you will be prioritising the care of your small group of patients. Usually this will be a group of six to nine patients within a bay and perhaps some side rooms. This is one of the most important skills to develop. If you cannot prioritise, you will waste time and be inefficient. This will cause stress both to yourself and to your fellow team members, as well as causing potential harm to your patients. You will develop your own way of ensuring that you are efficient, but the following will help you to decide what to do and when.

1   Decide if there is any urgent action that you need to take straight away. For example, if one of your patients is critically unwell you may need to record an electrocardiogram (ECG), give analgesia, record vital signs, administer oxygen and contact the doctors.

2   If your patients are stable following report, the first thing that you must do is go and introduce yourself to them. This has many functions. You will be able to see that your patients are how you expect them to be from the information given during report. Your patients will know who is looking after them for that shift. If a patient has become suddenly unwell, you will know straight away at the beginning of your shift. You will have the opportunity to discuss with the HCA or student with whom you are working the care that is required for each patient. This ensures that you both know what your responsibilities are for that shift. It also promotes good teamwork.

3   Your next job should be to assist your colleagues in getting the patients ready for breakfast (if you are on an early shift). This should not be left to the HCA/student to struggle on with while you 'grab' the drug trolley. It is very important that the patients' nutritional needs are met and that they are comfortable.

4   You must ensure that the patients' vital signs are measured and recorded before the medications are administered. This may be something that you have the time to do yourself, or else you could delegate it to an appropriate member of the team. You must know what the patient's observations are before giving cardiac drugs, for example. It will be too late if you have given a beta-blocker and then find out that the patient has a pulse of 40 beats/minute. What will your defence be if you are asked why you did not check the pulse before giving the drug when bradycardia is caused by beta-blockers? You would have *no* defence. 'The ward was too busy' is no excuse.

5   Now you can go and get the drug trolley! You will see other nurses doing this straight away following report, but when would they have done the above? The answer is they won't have – they will have expected someone else to do it. When you have ensured that your patients are safe and comfortable, you can concentrate on administering their medications. Because you have assisted your colleague in preparing the patients and making them comfortable, you will be less likely to be interrupted during the drug round. It is important that you are able to give this your full attention, especially when you are newly qualified, as interruptions can make it more likely that you will make a mistake. If you are responsible for side rooms as well as a bay of patients, it is a good idea to commence the drug round there. This is because you may not get to the side rooms for some time if you start in the bay, and therefore there may be a relatively long period of time during which the patients in the side rooms are not being observed.

6   Now life becomes more complicated. It is around this time that several things are happening on the ward at once. There may be doctors arriving to do their rounds, telephone calls from relatives start to intrude on your time, patients require assistance with their hygiene needs, multidisciplinary meetings may be happening, if you allow open visiting then visitors may be wanting to discuss their loved ones with you, commodes are required, tea rounds are due, drips require changing, and fluid/food charts need to be completed! Oh no! Where do you start? First, the key to good teamwork between yourself and the HCA/student with whom you are working is *communication*. Discuss who is doing what, and if you find yourself preoccupied for prolonged periods with any of the above-mentioned activities, talk to each other. Tell the HCA/student that you will be with them as soon as you can, and make sure that they

are OK. You can do little about telephone calls and relatives – this is where you need to keep conversations brief and to the point, or if the relative is going to be visiting for a while, ask if you could catch up with them later. Try to attend doctors' rounds. There are many reasons why this is so important, as we discussed in Chapter 2.

7   As activities crop up, you need to decide what your priorites are. Do you need to do something this morning, or can it wait until the patients' washes have been completed? Documentation is very important and should be done as soon as possible after the event. However, doctors' rounds and meetings can be documented later.

8   Finally, remember that good prioritising skills do not develop overnight. They take years of fine tuning and practice to get right. So don't be disheartened if you make the wrong choice between tasks – this is how you will learn. Ask others who you feel prioritise well what they would have done in the same situation.

Appropriate delegation

This will be a difficult skill for you, especially at first. You will need to get to know the other staff before you will feel truly comfortable delegating to others in the team. You may feel guilty about asking others to do tasks which you feel that you should be doing yourself.

What you need to realise (early on if you want to stay sane!) is that you can't possibly do everything yourself and that you will need to work as a team in order to deliver good patient care.

You may well feel that you can't ask others, especially HCAs who have worked on the ward for years, to do things for you. You will probably feel self-conscious and embarrassed.

The answer is that it's not what you ask them to do that is important – it's *how you ask them*. Good communication is the key to successful delegation. Take a few minutes to discuss with the HCA/student with whom you are working who will be doing what during that shift. Share the workload and be realistic. Don't overload yourself with care you don't really think you can give. The member of staff would rather know what their workload is at the beginning of the shift so that they can organise their time effectively. If you have to ask them to take on extra work during the shift, they will find this difficult. Keep communicating with them during the shift, and if you are held up with relatives or an acutely ill patient, tell them and explain that you will try to help them as soon as possible.

When you are delegating, always ensure that this is appropriate. It is your responsibility to ensure that the member of staff to whom you delegate is competent to perform the task. Although they are *responsible*, you remain *accountable*. For example, you cannot assume that the HCA/student with whom you are working is competent in the skill of measuring and recording a patient's blood pressure. Just because the member of staff has worked on that ward for a period of time, this does not mean that they have been taught correctly, if at all. You must assess their competence to perform the task before you allow them to do this independently. You can then justify your delegation of that skill if necessary.

Time management

This tends to go hand in hand with good prioritisation skills. Get these right and you will probably be able to manage your time well. However, this may not always be the case. You may have prioritised very well but still end up staying late to complete your documentation.

The key is not to try and do everything at once. If you know that you will have a relatively 'quiet' period after lunch, then do your writing then. You will be less likely to make a mistake and will also have time to carry out any other jobs that arise from doing the paperwork. For example, you may need to refer a patient to one of the multidisciplinary team and this may become apparent when you are completing the documentation for the doctors' rounds. If you try to do all of this in between caring for your patients, you are likely to make a mistake or forget to do it completely.

A common time-management error concerns breaks. You may be brilliant at ensuring that those working with you get theirs, but how about you? This is not unique to newly qualified nurses – you will see many nurses who have been qualified for years not taking their breaks. Sometimes this is unavoidable. For example, in an emergency situation you may find that you just don't have the chance. However, you must ensure that you take your break on more 'normal' days. It is very important to take time away from the ward area to recap on the shift so far and relax. It gives you the opportunity to socialise with your colleagues and talk about topics other than work. You will also have the chance to eat something! How can you give your best to your patients if your blood sugar level is low and you have eaten nothing all day? There is a common trend among nurses to be martyrs. We have all heard nurses saying things like 'Oh, I'll be OK, you go and have your lunch' or 'I never get any lunch, there's never any time'. On some occasions this may be true, but on most days there is no reason not to take your break. A good manager will insist on it! Remember that it is your break – so no paperwork or other jobs should go with you!

Flexibility in emergencies

During an emergency situation all members of staff must remain flexible in order to ensure that all patients are cared for. It is easy to become drawn into the emergency even if you are not required. It is exciting and different, and human nature draws us to such situations. However, remember that there are possibly more than 20 other patients to be cared for.

If the individual concerned is your patient, obviously you must be involved, as you know the most about the patient and their family. If the patient is not under your direct care, you will need to think about how you can care for your own patients and help with the nursing of the patients in the care of the nurse whose patient is unwell. This nurse will be concentrating on this one patient and their relatives. It is a great help if he/she does not have to worry about the drug round, observations and essential care of the other patients. This is what you can do.

1   Ensure that your own patients are settled and cared for. Ask the member of staff with whom you are working to carry on with caring for those patients while you offer your assistance to the other nurse.
2   Ask the nurse whose patient is unwell what he/she needs help with. This may be help with the acutely ill patient, or he/she may be worried about not having given medications to the rest of the patients, in which case you could do this for him/her.
3   The nurse whose patient is unwell may be concerned about the welfare of the other patients in that bay. You may be able to talk to them and allay their worries about what is going on. Remember to be honest with them. Don't tell them that the patient is all right if he/she is not. But also remember that you need to maintain confidentiality.

4   The nurse may need help with the relatives of the unwell patient. You may be able to offer a cup of tea and a listening ear while they are waiting for news. The nurse may need someone to look for the relatives coming on to the ward. There is nothing worse than family members arriving and walking into an arrest situation. Someone will need to stop them and explain what is going on.

During a shift where there is an emergency, you will never feel as if you have 'caught up'. This is something you must learn to accept. Those involved will need time to gather their thoughts, and often cannot just carry on as normal following an arrest. Make sure that your patients are safe and cared for, but do not worry if other jobs such as restocking the trolleys or making referrals have not been done. They can be done by the next shift of nurses. You will probably go home feeling as if you have not given your best to your patients that day, and if the outcome of the arrest was fatal, you will probably feel upset as well. Most nurses will feel this way, but remember that you have done your best in very difficult circumstances. How many other professions require you to give life-saving skills one minute, give bad news to a relative the next, and then do a tea round? Some days will be better than others, and you will learn to cope with these feelings as you become more experienced, although you will probably never overcome them. In a way it is a shame if you do, as you may have lost some of your empathy along the way.

Budgeting

Although this is not something that you will be directly involved in, you will have a huge part to play indirectly. The ward manager will be given a budget which he/she will be required to manage. This will include staffing costs and consumables, such as dressings and giving sets. Your role is to be aware of what you are using and of wastage. Think about what you take into contaminated side rooms. Anything that is not used will have to be thrown away. Just take in what you need, otherwise you will be wasting money. If you are involved in off-duty planning, look at the skill mix carefully in order to avoid unnecessary booking of extra staff. You may find that one day you have too many staff and another day not enough, necessitating extra staff and therefore extra money.

General finance

It is a good idea to be aware of the global situation and not just the situation of your ward with regard to finances. By this I mean that you should think about the national issues such as Government initiatives which usually have an impact on NHS funding. Also keep up to date with the financial position within your Trust. What cost improvement programmes have been implemented? What impact do hospital ratings have on the funds given to your Trust? These will have implications for your day-to-day work. For example, one cost improvement programme issue may be the use of agency staff. Your Trust may decide that agency nurses can only be used in specified circumstances. This may affect the numbers of nurses on your shift. Hospital ratings look at issues such as waiting times. This will impact on the pressure that you are under to discharge patients earlier and in a timely way. This will free up beds to enable elective patients to be admitted to meet waiting times and for patients waiting in Accident and Emergency and Assessment Units to be admitted within the specified time limit. The Trust will be penalised if they do not meet this target. When you begin to think about applying for more senior positions, you will need to have an overall knowledge of these issues as you may be asked about them in interview. Even if you are not asked, it will be obvious from the way you answer questions that you have a good knowledge of the Trust business.

Lost bed days

Due to the pressures on the NHS, we are required to ensure that patients receive the best care in a timely fashion. This does not mean scrimping on excellent care, but making sure that patients are discharged as soon as possible. If discharge planning is commenced on admission, potential problems are highlighted, ensuring that there is enough time to solve them, while not delaying the patient's discharge. Delayed discharges mean not only lost bed days, but also distress to the patient – very few patients actually like being in hospital! Delays also mean the potential for opportunistic infections to delay the patient's discharge further. All of this adds up to avoidable wastage of NHS money which could otherwise be spent on patient care. Sometimes there is little that nurses can do to aid the situation. For example, a patient may be waiting for a nursing-home place and funding may be a problem. There is then no alternative to keeping the patient in hospital where they can be cared for until they are able to go to their new home. This can be frustrating for the patient, their nurses and family. The important point to make here is not to make the patient feel as if they are not welcome and that they shouldn't be there. You may hear derogatory terms such as 'bed blockers' being used. This is unacceptable and unprofessional. These patients require nursing care and that is what is important.

Staff management

You may be required to 'practise' this on occasions during your first year. Although you will probably not be left in charge intentionally, there may be occasions when, for example, the senior nurse is sick. The managers within your unit will try to ensure that you are not in charge by moving someone from another ward to help, but sometimes this is not possible.

If you find yourself in this situation, *don't panic*! Remember that you are not the only nurse on duty. You will need to discuss the management of the patients and ensure that they are all cared for during your shift. If your managers cannot provide you with a more senior member of staff, ask for an extra HCA to take the pressure off and free you up to concentrate on running the ward. Remember that there is always someone more senior to ask – except if you are the Director of Nursing! If you are not sure, ask. If you feel out of your depth with an acutely ill patient, contact your manager again and complete the appropriate documentation to indicate this. It may be possible to move the patient to an area with more senior staff, or this may prompt the manager to rethink moving someone more senior to your ward. Don't forget the specialist nurses. Do you have a critical care or practice development nurse whom you could call upon to come and help you?

Off-duty planning

Although you probably won't have to actually write this, it is a good idea to gain a working knowledge of it and how difficult it is! This will make you more accepting of a 'bad' shift pattern or not getting all of your requested shifts. With a ward of possibly 30 staff, giving everyone exactly what they want is impossible. Added to the fact that some staff work part-time or do set shifts, staff need study time and annual leave. There are several things you can do to help the member of staff who has this responsibility. First, get your requests in early. There is nothing more frustrating than having finished the off duty and having someone say 'Oh, I forgot to write in that I really need that day off.' Be realistic about the amount of requests that you make. Try to make them only if they are really necessary. If you are requesting annual leave, take note of how many others are asking to be off at the same time as you. There will probably be a limit to the number of staff nurses who are allowed off at any one time. This can be very difficult during the summer months in particular. Also, this may sound obvious, but remember to take all of your annual leave entitlement! Some people get to the end of the financial year with weeks left over. If you have a kind ward manager, they may let you carry some over – otherwise you will lose it. So be careful. It is your responsibility to ensure that you take your leave, not your ward manager's! Study leave will be negotiable, and this will usually depend on what course you want to do. Is it essential for the area you are working in? If so, you will usually be given a higher percentage of paid study time. If you know that you are going on a course, ensure that you indicate this in the request book so that the person doing the off duty knows not to put you on shift that day. You may have told your ward manager last month that you were going on a study day, but they have a lot to think about, so don't expect them to remember! Again, take responsibility!

Clinical supervision

If this has not been formally offered to you, you may need to discuss issues informally with someone. This may be a more senior colleague with whom you get on well either on your ward or in another area. You will find that the issues which you need to raise will have changed since you first qualified. Whereas when you were newly qualified you will have had issues regarding delegation and prioritising, you will now be thinking about taking charge and staffing issues. It is very important that you speak to someone on a regular basis to discuss these issues and explore your reactions and feelings. You will rarely have time to do this while working, and it is not something that should be squeezed into a five-minute break. If this is not something that is routinely offered, speak to your ward manager about the possibility. Don't be afraid to express your opinions and ideas. You may find that this is something your manager has been thinking about for a while but has not had the opportunity to develop. You may even be able to take on the organisation of this.

Consultants and their specialities

It is important to be informed about the consultants with whom you work and their specialities. Find out when they usually do their ward rounds and at what time. Most will do them at approximately the same times each week. This will enable you to be prepared with the information that they will need and to manage your time so that you are free to participate in the round.

The more you can develop a rapport with the consultants in your area, the easier you will find it to express your ideas and opinions about the patients in their care, especially if your opinion does not match theirs! They will respect your opinion and be able to discuss alternatives with you in a non-challenging way if they know you. Take the time to get to know them and develop a mutual respect. Your patients will benefit from this good working relationship and your job will be more satis-fying.

Clinical nurse specialists/lead nurses

There will be numerous specialist and lead nurses within your Trust. Find out who they are and how to contact them. They are always keen to teach and assist you with any related problems. They are knowledgeable in their speciality and a valuable resource for your development. Some may even be able to work clinically with you to develop your practice. This is really benefi-cial, as you will learn much more by actually doing it and having someone working alongside you. Practice development nurses are also able to assist you in your development. For example, you may have a real problem with prioritising your care. Ask them to work with you and give you some feedback about what you could do differently. Specialist and lead nurses are responsible for leading the service for that speciality within nursing, so they will have a strategic and operational viewpoint. This means that strategically they will be developing the service and linking with other services to ensure better patient care. Operationally they will be teaching, advising and evaluating the care given.

Consultant nurses

Depending on where these nurses work, they may or may not have their own caseload. They will work specifically within a speciality (e.g. diabetes or care of the older person). They will be responsible for implementing Government initiatives such as National Service Frameworks (NSFs) and developing the service for the patients within that speciality. They will work both within a Trust and with other outside agencies, such as other Trusts, the strategic health authority and the Workforce Development Confederation. They will be leading the service and developing it alongside nurses in ward areas.

Hospital bed management

Having first-hand experience of this job in the past, I can truthfully say that it is one of the hardest jobs in the hospital! Not only does no one want to talk to you, but you have the job of giving news to patients that they don't want to hear. It is the bed manager's responsibility to ensure that patients are moved through the hospital in an efficient manner. They will work between Accident and Emergency, GP referrals and the wards to place the patient in the most appropriate bed. The reason why no one wants to talk to you is that when the bed manager rings the ward it is usually to ask you about your discharge status and to give you a patient to fill empty beds as soon as possible. This means there is no let-up for you. However, if Accident and Emergency waiting times and waiting-list targets are to be met, this is what must happen. The bed manager may have to cancel elective admissions for the next day if there are no beds available both on the ward and in the intensive-care unit (ITU), as some patients require ITU following their elective surgery (e.g. aneurysm repair). This is a very difficult task to perform, especially if the patient has been cancelled at short notice before or has taken time off work in preparation. Unfortunately, the patient will often shout (and swear) at the person who gives them this news – they are understandably upset and frustrated, and they may take this out on the easiest person, namely the bed manager.

It is important to remember these points when dealing with the bed manager. They are doing an important job and are not there to make your life difficult. Understanding the pressures that they are under may change the way you feel about them!

Mentoring students

This may well be something that you are becoming more involved in. There is now a clause within the NMC *Code of Professional Conduct* (Nursing and Midwifery Council 2002) stating that it is the responsibility of all qualified nurses to teach students. They are after all our colleagues of tomorrow, so let's teach them correctly now. This may be daunting at first. You may feel that you only just know what *you* should be doing, let alone a student nurse! However, this is one of the best ways of realising how much you do actually know. Students can be very challenging, and this sometimes causes nurses to be defensive.

Remember to be honest with the student. If you don't know the answer to their question, tell them this. Ask them to research the answer and to come back and give feedback to you. The student will respect you much more if you are honest rather than trying to bluff your way through the situation. They will also realise that it is acceptable to admit when you don't know something and that *no one knows everything*. The day when a nurse thinks he/she knows everything is a very dangerous one.

You may be asked if you would like to attend a formal mentorship course. This will qualify you to assess students' practice. This is a very important process within the students' development. As a mentor you will be acting as a gatekeeper to the profession, ensuring high-quality newly qualified nurses (Department of Health 2001). You are responsible for ensuring that the nurses of tomorrow are competent.

When mentoring students there are key elements to remember, whether you are a qualified mentor or not.

• Make them feel welcome. This is the most important part of a student's experience, and it will colour their whole placement. Ensure that they have a ward student pack (if there is one – if not, you could develop one). Show them around the ward, tell them where the toilets are and where to go for their break, and so on. Show them that you were expecting them (even if you weren't!). Sometimes the university–Trust communication process could be better and students may turn up unexpectedly. If this happens, *bluff*!

- Make sure that you know where the student is in their development. Don't assume that because this is not their first ward they know how to measure and record vital signs competently. Conversely, don't assume that if it is their first ward they don't know anything. Make the time to sit down with them and agree a learning plan. Find out what they feel confident in and what skills they feel they need to develop further. Make a list of the skills they feel they lack, and try to accommodate the learning of these while they are with you.

- Ensure that the student is able to access learning opportunities. As they have supernumerary status, they should be able to access opportunities as they arise, not just if they are not busy. For example, if a patient is going to another hospital for an investigation, the student should be allowed to attend with them to observe and learn about something that is not offered within their Trust. They may never get this opportunity again. This is the true meaning of supernumerary status – it does not mean that the student should not be involved in patient care and with the workload of the ward, but that they should not miss out on learning because of it.

- Be honest with your student. They will appreciate both positive and negative feedback, so remember to give them both! Students need to know what they do well and what requires improvement, otherwise they will not develop. Learn to give constructive criticism. If you have serious concerns about your student, do something about it! This sounds obvious, but often mentors give the student the benefit of the doubt and think that the next mentor will pick up the problem. This is very dangerous and can mean a student being failed during their last placement for something that should have been picked up months ago, or alternatively qualifying when they are not competent. It is not fair on either the student or future mentors not to say anything. More importantly, it is part of your code of conduct to ensure that any concerns are made known and acted upon. This is extremely difficult to do, and can be very upsetting for both the mentor and the student. First ask another member of the team to work with the student to ensure that your assessment is valid. If they agree, now is the time to involve the student's tutor and/or the person responsible for students within the Trust. They will support you and the student and initiate an action plan. This gives you a process to work through with the student and specific objectives for them to meet. In most cases, if this is done early on the student will be able to progress and will thank you for highlighting these areas of development. Unfortunately, on rare occasions the student is unable to perform at the required level, and for the safety of the patients must be failed in practice. If you have the misfortune to be involved in this, it is likely to be one of the most difficult things you have ever had to do. You must always ask yourself 'Would I want this nurse caring for a loved one of mine?' If the answer is no, then you must do something about it. It is your professional responsibility to do so. Thankfully this is not a regular occurrence, but it is what mentors are there for.

7

The future

Keeping yourself up to date

It is a requirement of the Nursing and Midwifery Council as identified within *The PREP Handbook* (Nursing and Midwifery Council 2001) that you meet the following requirements.

- You must have completed a minimum of 100 days (750 hours) of practice within the 5 years prior to renewal of registration.
- You must have undertaken at least 5 days (35 hours) of learning activity *relevant to your area of practice* in the 3 years prior to the renewal of your registration. This must be recorded within your professional profile. This profile may be requested upon renewal as evidence.
- Examples of learning activities include the following:
  - reflection with regard to learning that has taken place informally or formally within the workplace
  - in-house or university-based study days/courses; certificate and reflection of learning that has taken place
  - library work – you may have spent time researching a subject relevant to your work; summary of research and impact on your work
  - regular reading of nursing and medical journals; keeping a reading log of what you have learned and any changes in practice as a result of it

- keeping up to date with media coverage of nursing issues
- attending conferences.

Extended roles

During your first year you may have the chance to take on extra responsibilities and extend your role. Before you agree to this, ensure that you are ready. For example, are you confident in your ability to administer oral drugs before you consider taking on the responsibility of administering intravenous drugs? You may feel under pressure to take on these roles, but if you don't feel ready you must say so. The period when you are newly qualified is stressful enough without taking on more than you can comfortably cope with. When you decide that you are ready, the following are some of the roles that you may consider.

- *Mentor preparation.* (Most universities stipulate that you must be 1 year post registration to apply for this course.) This role is very important both for your development and for the learning environment within which you are working. It is essential that there are sufficient mentors within each clinical placement to effectively mentor the students of the future. After all, they will be your colleagues one day. This course may be asked for when you are applying for more senior posts.
- *Venepuncture.* This is a valuable skill to obtain, as you will be able to provide a more efficient service for your patients. For example, if your patient is due to be discharged that day and they are being discharged while taking anticoagulant therapy, their discharge may be dependent on their clotting times and you may realise that your patient has not

had blood taken that day. You will then be able to take the blood sample and not have to wait for a doctor to come and take it, which could delay the discharge for hours.

- *Cannulation*. Again this is a very valuable skill to have. Nurses are formally taught this skill to avoid infection and damage to the veins. You will be able to evaluate the cannula in place for patency, and to replace it in a timely manner if necessary. You would not need to wait for a doctor to be free, which could mean a delay in a patient receiving important drugs intravenously.

- *Intravenous drug administration*. This is now commonly seen as a nurse's job, but 10 years ago it was most definitely part of a doctor's role. This shows how over a relatively short period of time tasks and responsibilities can shift from one profession to another. The nurse must ensure that he/she feels confident about and is competent to take on this role and understands related issues such as anaphylaxis. Practice mixing and drawing up the drugs now, as this will help you when you come to undertake this course.

- *Male recatheterisation*. Again, this helps to ensure the patient's comfort and enhances their care. A patient who requires a new catheter will not want to wait very long before a new one is inserted! If the nurse has undertaken the appropriate training, he/she will be able to care for the patient in this way without the need to wait. This also helps to ensure the holistic care of the patient.

As you progress through your career, there may be other extended roles that you wish to take on. Remember that you must feel ready and not pressurised into this, and if you are taking on more and more roles, what is happening to the fundamentals of the nurse's role – the essential nursing care? Are those who are doing this appropriately trained and supervised? Are you willing to give this up?

Individual performance reviews (IPR)/appraisals

These should take place regularly, usually once a year. This is an opportunity for you to spend valuable time with your manager and discuss your progress. You will have the chance to discuss areas that you would like to develop – for example, courses that you would like to attend. Your manager will be able to offer constructive feedback about your performance over the past year. There should be no great surprises here – if a manager has concerns about your performance, they should be addressed at the time, and not wait for the IPR. However, they may identify areas that could be improved – for example, your organisational skills.

If any areas are identified, try not to be defensive but to see this as an opportunity to learn from others and develop your practice. It is more likely that you will be praised for your work over the past year and discussions on how to progress through your chosen career will be explored. If you want to progress to a more senior position, your manager will be able to offer guidance on how to do this. Remember that not everyone wants to 'climb the ladder'. It is OK not to want to do this. For some nurses it is important that they remain at the front-line ensuring excellent patient care, while others want to be part of the management of that care. Both are very important parts to play.

The most valuable part of the IPR process is to receive feedback and to realise that you are appreciated and a valuable member of the team.

Sharing your knowledge

You will find that now you are qualified, you will be required to teach many different levels of staff. This may be a new healthcare assistant, a student nurse, a new staff nurse or any other type of learner that may be present on the ward. You will also be required to teach junior doctors when they first qualify. You will find that their level of practical knowledge will be limited in the first few months.

Teaching is a privilege that we as nurses enjoy on a day-to-day basis. One of the most satisfying parts of nursing is passing on what you have learnt. Teaching can take place anywhere – the patient's bedside, the clinical room, in hand-over and during meetings, for example.

You may also be asked if you would like to teach in a more formal setting, for example during healthcare assistant induction. This is an excellent way to start teaching, especially if you are not confident in this type of situation.

One-to-one teaching

Teaching whilst in the ward environment will probably be one-to-one and spontaneous. There will be little preparation required and it will be a subject that you are likely to be confident in, as it is probably part of your everyday nursing.

Try to ensure that you have enough time to teach the skill/subject you are intending. There is nothing more annoying for both you and the learner than being constantly interrupted, although this cannot always be helped.

• Before beginning the session, you will need to check the learner's prior experience regarding the subject. This is important in order to build upon the learner's existing knowledge. If you are teaching a skill, you could ask the learner to show you what they know already.

- Ensure that the equipment you need is to hand. You will not want to be going in and out of the room to get items you have forgotten.
- Whilst teaching check regularly the learner's understanding. This will ensure that you do not loose their attention. Make sure the learner can see what you are doing and encourage them to ask questions as you go along.
- When you have finished your session, summarise the content of the session and ask for any questions.
- Ask for feedback on your teaching style and for some evaluation of the session. This may be written or verbal.
- Ensure that you reinforce that the learner must not practice the skill if they do not feel competent and should ask to be shown again if this is the case.

Group teaching

- It is always best to write a lesson plan for formal teaching. This will help you to plan the session and keep to time. Remember though, this must be flexible in order to respond to the needs of the learners. Within the plan, include an introduction to the session, the various elements of the subject and a conclusion.
- Ensure the environment is conducive to teaching *and* learning. The room should be of a comfortable temperature – too hot and the learners may fall asleep, too cold and they will not be able to concentrate! Try to make sure it is quiet, you may need to shut doors and windows – again lots of noise will distract both you and the learner. If it is within your power, provide some refreshments for the beginning of the session or at the break if there is one. This will make the learners feel valued and worthwhile. It will also make you and them feel more relaxed

and you will have the chance to chat to them.

- Ensure you discuss 'housekeeping' – where the toilets are, fire procedures, break times and tidying up after themselves!
- If you are planning to use teaching aids, ensure you know how to work them before the session. Using different teaching aids and styles will help to keep your learners' attention. For example, overhead projectors, computers, written information, practical demonstration and discussion.
- Almost all teaching concerned with nursing can be practical as well as theoretical. Your learners will enjoy the session much more if they can be interactive and are not just listening to you talk. You will also find it more enjoyable.
- If you do not know the members of the group, start by introducing yourself and asking them to do the same. You can also plan an 'ice-breaker' to help the group feel more comfortable talking in front of each other, especially if they do not already know one another. A good place to find some interesting ice-breakers is on the Internet – you will find some unusual ones! A word of warning – don't choose really embarrassing ones as you will lose the confidence of the group.
- Outline the aims of the session and check that what you are about to teach them is what they are expecting! I was once asked to teach at very short notice a group of healthcare assistants. I had no time to prepare so was forced to use a previous teacher's teaching material. I was told that the subject was Basic Observations and MEWS (Modified Early Warning System). This was a subject that I felt confident in teaching, having done it many times before. When I started the session, I checked the healthcare assistants' previous knowledge and it transpired that they were all from outside the Trust – from nursing homes, GP surgeries, etc. I had planned

to teach them about using the hospital monitors and about MEWS. This was obviously going to be of no use to them whatsoever! I then had to think on my feet and decide how I was going to fill the next 2 hours.

Golden rules!

- If you don't know the answer to a question that may be asked during a session, don't try to bluff your way through it. It will probably be obvious that you are not really sure of your answer, and you could lose your credibility. Admit that you don't know and explore the possible answers together. Not only will this identify you as someone who is open and honest, but will reinforce to the learners that it is OK not to know everything!
- Keep eye contact with the learner/s. It is easy to concentrate too much on the overhead projector or your notes. This is not a good way to conduct a session, as you will not keep the learner's interest.
- When teaching more than one learner, ensure that you make eye contact with all members of the group. You may already know one of the members of the group and feel more comfortable talking to them. This will make the other members of the group feel like 'outsiders', making them less likely to interact.
- Try to accommodate all styles of learning. Remember that some learners will be more comfortable with 'chalk and talk', others with more interactive styles such as role play. This way you will engage all members of the group and allow them to participate when they feel most comfortable.
- Be prepared! Don't use other people's material – handouts, OHPs or equipment – unless you have to. Ensure you know your subject well so that you can talk around the subject.

- Ensure that your information and research is up to date. Don't just use the same session time and time again without updating it. Eventually there will be a learner who will point this out to the group, which could be very embarrassing.
- Be enthusiastic! This will take you a long way in teaching. Enjoy your subject, sound interested in it and always relate it back to real life on the wards.

8

Common clinical problems

The following is a guide to the most common problems you will encounter while working clinically. It is not exhaustive and is in no way a replacement for the vast amounts of knowledge to be accessed around you!

You may find that a patient will suddenly become unwell and present with a particular symptom. That symptom will be a clue to the underlying problem.

Assessing an acutely unwell patient (adapted from Smith 2003)

The following is a system for assessing an acutely unwell patient. Use steps A–E to help you to find out what is happening to your patient. This can be used in all emergency situations, including a collapsed patient or one whose condition has deteriorated due to an unknown reason. It is important to remember to *look* at your patient. Their vital signs may be misleading. For example, I was on a ward as a student nurse when the emergency call bell was activated. The staff rushed to commence basic life support, only to find the patient sitting up in bed reading a newspaper! The doctor who had activated the alarm had walked past and seen a 'flat line' on the monitor, and had not looked at the patient!

A Airway   Is it patent/partially obstructed/fully obstructed? If so, can the obstruction be removed (e.g. food)? Is the patient unconscious? If so, apply a Guedel airway.

B Breathing   Assess rate, rhythm, depth and effort. Do not rely on an oxygen saturation monitor, as this will only tell you the percentage of oxygen within the patient's blood, not the quality of their breathing.

Is the patient making sufficient effort on their own? If not, consider assisting with a bag, valve and mask. Do not wait for the patient to have a respiratory arrest – use the bag to complement the patient's own breaths. Ask an experienced nurse/practice development nurse to show you how to do this.

Look at the chest movements. Are they equal? If not, this could indicate a collapsed lung.

C Circulation   Feel the patient's skin. Is it dry, warm, cold or clammy?

Check the capillary refill time (CRT). This will indicate the state of the peripheral circulation.

Check the pulse for rate, rhythm and strength. Check the blood pressure, although this can often be a late sign of shock, especially in a young fit adult. This is because the body will compensate for some time by vasoconstricting the blood vessels in order to keep the blood pressure high enough to perfuse the major organs. Do not be fooled by a normal blood pressure.

D Disability   Check the blood glucose level, even if the patient is not a known diabetic.

Check the AVPU (Alert, Voice, Pain, Unresponsive) or the GCS (Glasgow Coma Score).

Check the pupils. Are they equal and reactive?

E Exposure   Finally, carry out a thorough examination of the patient. Look for wounds, infection and bleeding (internal/external).

Breathlessness

This procedure should be followed if the patient suddenly becomes more breathless than usual.

1 Measure and record the respiratory rate, rhythm, depth and effort. The normal rate is 12–14 per minute. Record other vital signs.
2 Measure and record the oxygen saturation. The normal range is 95–100%.
3 If the patient is known to be asthmatic, measure the peak flow if possible. Then compare the result with their normal average result.
4 Apply 100% oxygen via a non re-breathe mask. Inflate the bag first. In patients who may have carbon-dioxide-retaining problems this can be corrected later. Otherwise they will die first from lack of oxygen.
5 Call the doctor and inform them of the above findings and actions. Document everything.

Possible causes

- Myocardial infarction. Breathlessness may be due to infarction of part of the cardiac muscle, causing lack of oxygen in the blood and leading to increased respiratory rate. Chest pain would usually be present, but this is not always so.

- Pulmonary embolus. Increased respiratory rate is due to blockage of a pulmonary artery, usually by a blood clot, causing lack of blood supply to the lungs, leading to increased respiratory rate in order to compensate. Chest pain and cyanosis may also be present.
- Pneumothorax. Breathlessness is due to an accumulation of air within the pleural space resulting in lack of available oxygen in the blood. There is unequal air entry heard via a stethoscope, as well as unilateral movement of the chest wall.
- Pulmonary oedema. Breathlessness is due to fluid overload, which results in inability of the lungs to absorb oxygen.
- Pneumonia. Breathlessness is caused by exudate produced in the presence of infection. This obstructs the airways, leading to an increased respiratory rate.
- Anaphylaxis. This is due to an adverse reaction, usually to a drug or type of food. Airway constriction due to bronchospasm and oedema causes lack of oxygen supply to the lungs and breathlessness.

Chest pain

This procedure should be followed if the patient develops sudden chest pain.

1 Record vital signs.
2 Record oxygen saturation level.
3 Apply 100% oxygen (as before).
4 Assess the type and location of pain. If the patient is known to have angina and glyceryltrinitrate (GTN) is prescribed, administer sub-lingually.

5 Inform the doctor of the above.
6 Record an ECG.

Possible causes

- Angina. Lack of blood supply to the cardiac muscle is caused by atherosclerosis. This leads to lack of oxygen supply to the muscle, causing pain.
- Myocardial infarction (MI). Lack of oxygen supply to the cardiac muscle is caused by blockage of blood supply to the muscle, leading to tissue damage and pain (although some MIs can be 'silent' and cause little or no pain). Pain is often felt in the left arm, chest and throat, and it is often described as crushing.
- Pulmonary embolus. Pain is caused by lack of oxygen supply to the cardiac muscle, due to blockage of the pulmonary artery.
- Musculoskeletal causes. Pain is often due to straining of the chest wall muscles or ribs. Often the patient will feel pain when the rib is pressed.
- Gastric causes. Gastritis can cause chest pain due to inflammation, and is often accompanied by reflux.
- Dissecting aortic aneurysm. Pain is due to loss of fluid from the aorta, which leads to lack of blood supply to the heart muscles. Typically patients will show large discrepancies in their blood pressure between the right and left arms. A difference of 40 mmol may indicate this.

Abdominal pain

This procedure should be followed if the patient suddenly complains of severe abdominal pain.

1   Record vital signs.
2   Dipstick test the urine for blood and protein.
3   Check the bowel history.
4   Allow nothing by mouth.
5   Inform the doctor of the above.

Possible causes

- Constipation. Patients may experience severe pain if they are very constipated. This may be accompanied by flatulence and repeated requests for the toilet. They may have a distended abdomen.
- Adhesions. If your patient has had recent surgery, adhesions may have been caused.
- Obstruction. This will be accompanied by the absence of bowel sounds or motion, and by vomiting and distension.
- Urinary tract infection or retention. Check for the presence of a palpable bladder.

Oliguria

This procedure should be followed if the patient has poor/no urine output.

1   Record hourly urine measurements. The minimum acceptable output is 30 ml/hour.
2   Record vital signs.
3   Check for the presence of a palpable bladder.
4   Check the most recent blood results for indications of dehydration/renal failure.
5   Inform the doctor of the above.

Possible causes

- Hypovolaemia. This may be caused by dehydration, bleeding or cardiac failure. Lack of circulating volume causes low blood pressure and renal failure.
- Drug toxicity. This is due to drugs which are nephrotoxic (e.g. penicillin, non-steroidal anti-inflammatory drugs).
- Sepsis.
- Blocked catheter. This sounds obvious, but check before calling the doctor! A simple bladder washout could cure the problem. If the catheter is blocked with debris or thick urine, obtain a catheter specimen of urine (CSU).

Neurological deterioration

This procedure should be followed if the patient shows a sudden deterioration in their neurological condition.

1 Check the airway and ensure its patency. If the patient is unconscious, apply a Guedel airway. Administer 100% oxygen.
2 Check the patient's breathing (rate, depth, effort and rhythm). Assist their breathing with bag, valve and mask if necessary.
3 Check the circulation (pulse, blood pressure, skin colour/warmth/clamminess). Check the patient's temperature.
4 Check the AVPU/GCS. Check for equal, reactive pupils.
5 Check the blood glucose level.
6 Examine the patient for obvious causes (e.g. recent surgery, blood loss, septicaemia, severe cellulitis).
7 Inform the doctor of the above.

Possible causes

- Dehydration. Severe dehydration can cause drowsiness and confusion. Check fluid input and urine output. Examine skin integrity, as dry, inelastic skin can indicate dehydration.
- Cerebral event. This may be a bleed or infarct. Loss of motor ability, consciousness level, speech and bladder/ bowel function as well as confusion may be an indication. Look at the pupils. They should be of equal size and reactive.
- Toxicity. This can be due to drugs or infection. Examine the drug chart for drugs which are known to cause drowsiness/confusion. Check for possible infection and pyrexia.
- Don't forget unusual causes such as Guillain-Barré's syndrome.

Confusion

This procedure should be followed if the patient becomes suddenly confused.

1 Check the blood glucose level.
2 Dipstick test the urine for blood and protein.
3 Check vital signs.
4 Check the oxygen saturation level. If it is below 95% and the patient is co-operative, administer 100% oxygen.
5 Inform the doctor of the above.

Possible causes

- Acute exacerbation of an existing condition (e.g. dementia or other psychiatric disorder). Examine the patient's history and any drugs that they may be taking which would indicate this.

- Metabolic causes, such as a high level of sodium or potassium. Look at the patient's most recent blood results.
- Hypoxia. Check the saturation levels. This will only be a guide – remember that the true values will only be seen when arterial blood is taken for analysis.
- Drug toxicity. Check the drug chart for known drugs that may cause confusion (e.g. opiates).
- Infections. Most commonly these are urinary tract infections, which can be easily treated with antibiotics.
- Neurological causes (e.g. cerebrovascular accident, transient ischaemic attack). Usually accompanied by other signs such as loss of motor control and slurred speech.
- Post-operatively. The patient may become confused following surgery (e.g. due to hypoxia, hypovolaemia, dehydration, medications or anaesthetic drugs).
- Alcohol withdrawal. This is commonly observed on the third day of admission. Always check the patient's usual intake. They may not consider it to be high, but their body may be used to it. If a high intake is suspected, consider the use of withdrawal drugs prophylactically, as this is preferable to having to deal with an aggressive, confused patient.

Seizures

This procedure should be followed if the patient collapses with signs of seizure.

1 Protect the airway. Place the patient in the recovery position if possible.
2 Reassure the patient and stay with them. Do not try to restrain them.
3 Most seizures last less than 5 minutes, but if they are prolonged, administer 100% oxygen to prevent hypoxia.

4 Check the blood glucose level.
5 Inform the doctor of the above.

Possible causes

- Epilepsy. The patient may be a known epileptic, in which case sedatives may be prescribed as required.
- Head injury/cerebral event. Cerebral oedema may cause irritation and seizures.
- Drug/alcohol withdrawal.
- Febrile convulsions. Seizures are sometimes seen in children, due to fever and hypoxia.
- Drug overdose. Typically seizures are caused by psychiatric drugs.
- Metabolic causes (e.g. hypoglycaemia).

Haematemesis/per rectum (PR) bleeding

This procedure should be followed if the patient is losing fresh blood per rectum or vomiting.

1 Measure the amount of blood lost.
2 Ensure that there is a cannula *in situ.*
3 Measure the vital signs. Remember that low blood pressure is often a late sign of hypovolaemic shock. Record lying and standing blood pressures if the patient's condition will allow this. A difference in these readings will indicate to you whether a significant amount of blood has been lost. Concentrate more on the pulse and respiratory rate. Note the skin temperature, clamminess and capillary refill time (CRT).
4 Ensure that IV fluids are given if these have been prescribed.

5 Administer 100% oxygen.
6 Reassure the patient.
7 Give prescribed anti-emetic if the patient is vomiting.
8 Inform the doctor of the above.

Note: A word on monitors! Although they are very useful when you are treating an acutely ill patient, monitors must be used with caution. Most vital signs monitors are not designed for recording routine observations from patient to patient. This is because they do not always recalibrate themselves between patients, especially if the machine has not been switched off between patients. This may result in inaccurate readings. They are most useful when you need to monitor a patient's vital signs closely (e.g. every 15 minutes). If you are using a monitor in this way, ensure that you set the parameters individually for that particular patient.

This will ensure that an alarm sounds if the vital signs fall outside these parameters. If you have done this and the alarm sounds, return to the patient and find out what is happening. All too often an alarm is sounding and the nurses do not take any notice.

Be cautious when you are using these machines to record pulse. They will not always detect a tachycardia, and certainly will not identify rhythm. You will also not know the strength of the pulse. For example, you may be misled into thinking that the pulse is 70 beats/minute, when in fact it is 160 beats/minute, irregular and weak.

While you are caring for your acutely ill patient, remember that you are part of a team – involve colleagues and doctors, and document everything.

Checklist

Objective	Achieved	Date
Pre-qualification Management/supervised practice		
Allocation and delegating skills		
Management of a group of patients		
Doctors' rounds and case conferences		
Drug rounds		
Off-duty planning and staffing issues		
Ordering of supplies		
Use of the computer		
Sisters' meetings		
Knowledge of policies and procedures		
Your first day post qualification		
Cardiac arrest procedures		
Fire evacuation and procedures		
The first few weeks		
Case conferences		
Taking charge of your group of patients		
Fundamental nursing care		
Undertaking a ward round		
Patient admission		

Objective	Achieved	Date
What to do in the event of a death		
Ward philosophy of care		
Doctors' rota		
Nursing rota		
Senior nurse support		
Working on the nurse 'bank' or doing extra shifts		
Electronic equipment		
Important policies		
The next two to six weeks		
When to contact doctors		
Preparation for theatre/investigations		
Post-operative care		
Nasogastric tubes		
PEG tubes		
Enteral feeding		
Urinary catheterisation		
Blood transfusions		
Referrals		
Your first year		
Prioritising acute care		
Appropriate delegation		
Time management		

Objective	Achieved	Date
Flexibility in emergencies		
Budgets		
General finance		
Lost bed days		
Staff management		
Off-duty planning		
Clinical supervision		
Consultants and their specialities		
Clinical nurse specialists/lead nurses		
Consultant nurses		
Hospital bed management		
Mentoring students		

References

Benner P (1984) *From Novice to Expert: excellence and power in professional nursing practice.* Addison-Wesley Publishing Company, London.

Department of Health (2001) *The Essence of Care.* Department of Health, London.

Department of Health (2001) *Preparation of Mentors and Teachers.* Department of Health, London.

Gibbs G (1988) *Learning by Doing: a guide to teaching and learning methods.* Oxford Polytechnic Further Education Unit, Oxford.

Nursing and Midwifery Council (2001) *The PREP Handbook.* Nursing and Midwifery Council, London.

Nursing and Midwifery Council (2002) *Code of Professional Conduct.* Nursing and Midwifery Council, London.

Nursing and Midwifery Council (2002) *Guidelines for the Administration of Medicines.* Nursing and Midwifery Council, London.

Smith G (2003) *ALERT – Acute Life Threatening Events: recognition and treatment.* University of Portsmouth, Portsmouth.

Stockwell F (1972) *The Unpopular Patient.* Croom Helm Ltd, London.

Index